The Brain Code

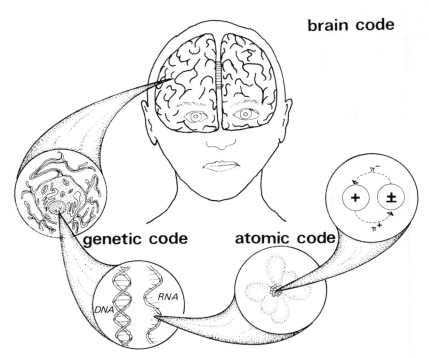

Frontispiece The codes of nature.

The Brain Code

MECHANISMS OF INFORMATION TRANSFER
AND THE ROLE OF THE CORPUS CALLOSUM

Norman D. Cook

WOLFSON COLLEGE, OXFORD

METHUEN
London and New York

First published in 1986 by
Methuen & Co. Ltd
11 New Fetter Lane, London EC4P 4EE

Published in the USA by
Methuen & Co.
in association with Methuen, Inc.
29 West 35th Street, New York NY 10001

Photoset by Rowland Phototypesetting Ltd
Bury St Edmunds, Suffolk
Printed in Great Britain

British Library Cataloguing in Publication Data
Cook, Norman D.
 The brain code: mechanisms of information
 transfer and the role of the corpus
 callosum.
 1. Brain   2. Psychology, Physiological
 I. Title
 612'.82   QP376
 ISBN 0-416-40840-0

Library of Congress Cataloging in Publication Data
Cook, Norman D.
 The brain code.

 Includes index.
 1. Corpus callosum.   2. Brain—Localization of
functions.   3. Laterality.   4. Neuropsychology.
I. Title.
QP382.2.C66   1986   612'.82   86–8368
ISBN 0-416-40840-0

Contents

Tables and figures

Tables

Figures

viii

Acknowledgments

Acknowledgment is made to the following for permission to reproduce or adapt copyrighted illustrations from the sources named:

Figure 2.2: adapted from R. Nieuwenhuys et al. (1978) *The Human Central Nervous System*, Berlin, Springer-Verlag. Figure 2.20: adapted from a paper by N. A. Lassen et al., *Scientific American*, October 1978. Figure 2.23: adapted from a paper by J. R. Wolff and L. Zaborsky (1979) in I. S. Russell et al. (eds), *Structure and Function of Cerebral Commissures*, New York, Macmillan. Figure 3.1: from a paper by P. S. Goldman-Rakic (1984) *Trends in the Neurosciences*, Nov., 419–24. Figures 3.2 and 3.4: from a paper by J. C. Hedreen and T. C. T. Yin (1981) *Journal of Comparative Neurology*, 197, 605–21. Figure 4.3: adapted from a paper by P. Rakic and P. I. Yakovlev (1968) *Journal of Comparative Neurology*, 132, 45–72. Figure 6.1: from a paper by E. G. Jones and T. P. S. Powell (1970) *Brain*, 93, 793–820. Figure 6.10: from a paper by D. E. Mitchell and C. Blackemore (1970) *Vision Research*, 10, 49–54. Figure A1.6 (A): adapted from a paper by L. E. White (1965) *International Review of Neurobiology*, 8, 1–34. Figure A1.8: adapted from a paper by L. W. Swanson (1983) in W. Seifert (ed.), *Neurobiology of the Hippocampus*, New York, Academic.

Many thanks also go to my wife, Sumiko, and son, Alex – who, among other things, modeled for figures 2.13 and 2.10 (respectively).

NORMAN D. COOK, 1986

Preface
WHAT IS THE 'BRAIN CODE'?

Phrases such as the 'brain code' are used to describe the set of fundamental rules concerning how information is stored and transmitted from site to site within the brain. Unlike the 'neuron code,' which is concerned with how individual neurons receive and transmit neural impulses, the 'brain code' is concerned with the mechanisms by which large groups of neurons transmit the images, thoughts and feelings which we suspect are the fundamental units of our psychological lives. Although a great deal is now known concerning the neuron code, relatively little is firmly established concerning the brain code. Even when it is possible to state that memory is lost when a certain part of the brain is damaged or that speech comprehension is impaired when a different area is destroyed, the underlying mechanisms of normal information transfer have remained unclear.

Ultimately most research in psychology and the neurosciences is aimed at the deciphering of the brain code – often by means of clarification of aspects of the neuron code, but normally the behavioral implications for the whole organism, rather than the strictly cellular implications, are the matters of primary concern. Yet, because of the many complexities of the human mind and brain and the apparent lack of understanding of fundamental issues, few psychologists would today embark on the writing of a treatise with a title as grandiose as 'The Brain Code.' Most would confess that the unraveling of the actual code is work for future generations and insist that important groundwork remains to be done.

Yet here we psychologists stand in one of the oldest fields of speculation, theorizing and experimental dabbling – still proclaiming that we are a 'young science'! To the contrary, not only do I think we work in an old and venerable field of enquiry with enough methodological care to qualify psychology as a science, but also I believe that sufficient groundwork on the brain code has in fact been completed and we can begin to construct some durable – if not yet elegant – theoretical edifices.

The perspective on brain function discussed in the following chapters is not claimed to be a complete unraveling of the brain code, but I do believe that it is the beginning of same and that the direction of future developments is already clearly indicated. Although many difficult and complex problems remain, a few fundamental and conceptually straightforward facts about brain function have emerged. As will be discussed at length, I believe that some of the most significant findings have been found in studies on the specializations of the cerebral hemispheres. Not only is hemispheric specialization itself an interesting topic – but also, more importantly, elucidation of how any two anatomically well-defined structures interact will inevitably have implications which extend far beyond the issue of 'hemisphericity' and 'dominance' and are likely to throw light on basic issues concerning the brain code. More than anything else, this contention that the hemisphere issue is *fundamental*, and not merely one of many fascinating subworlds of psychology, is perhaps the unique perspective of this book.

The proposed mechanism of information transfer which is developed in these chapters concerns the interaction of the two halves of bilateral animal nervous systems – particularly the means by which the cerebral hemispheres of the human brain communicate with one another across the corpus callosum. I argue that this interaction is analogous to the process of transcription between DNA and RNA within the cellular system – in other words, a fundamental 'control center' interaction which has influences on all other events in the system.

Although it might be said that nucleic acid transcription is the 'easy half' of the genetic code (since the translation process from nucleic acid to protein is both biochemically more complex and conceptually less obvious), it can equally be said that the problem of how 'translation' from gene to working protein occurs in the cell was reduced to one of finite dimensions with the discovery of transcription and an understanding of how the nucleic acids interact. Once the concept of nucleotide base-pairing became known, a small set of cryptographic possibilities for translating the 4-element nucleic acid code into the 22-element amino acid code was immediately apparent. In other words, the first and most important step in the deciphering of the 'genetic code' was the discovery of the fundamental interactions of the nucleic acids.

Similarly the proposed mechanism of *inter*hemispheric communication between the cerebral hemispheres is, in comparison with the complexities of *intra*hemispheric information processing within each hemisphere, uncomplicated and certainly the 'easy half' of the brain code. The *inter*hemispheric process is, however, important not only because it constitutes a high-level mechanism of information transfer, but also because it suggests a finite class of possibilities concerning how neural information may be transmitted *intra*hemispherically. Some discussion of those possibilities is made in chapter 8, but most of this area remains unexplored. The bulk of the book is concerned with demonstration of the nature of *inter*hemispheric communication and subsequently with arguments about the importance of hemispheric relations for our understanding of the 'brain code.'

My one qualifying note concerning this theory of the brain, however, is that none of the facts and discoveries which are essential ingredients in the brain code is as dramatic and unambiguous as the discoveries that led to the elucidation of the 'atomic code' and the 'genetic code.' Although the modern neurosciences have been able to provide a great deal of detailed knowledge upon which to build theories of brain function, the problem which the psychologist faces in constructing a theoretical framework is that there is in fact such a wealth of empirical findings – with no obvious 'elementary particles' or 'psychological genes' among them. Given the subject matter and the interest which the workings of the human mind have had for psychologists for many decades, this embarrassing abundance of empirical findings (the validity of each of which is often uncertain) is hardly surprising, but it does mean that the first steps toward 'deciphering the brain code' will be largely a conceptual achievement – the establishment of a hierarchy of importance among known facts and not the isolation of a royal molecule or the discovery of a surprise antic by a laboratory rat.

This is not to say that there are no explicit conclusions to be drawn from this theory of brain function nor to say that we are engaged in nothing more than tossing around an old philosophical chestnut, but the argument is, by its very nature, one which is more suggestive than conclusive – even when talking about new data and explicit predictions. In other words, brain code or no brain code, psychology is not metallurgy or applied genetics and the principal fruits of our labors are more likely to be conceptual than material.

The layout of the book is as follows: chapter 1 serves as a brief introduction to brain science and presents the basic arguments concerning the importance of the bilaterality of animal nervous systems. Here it is suggested that consideration of topics such as 'laterality' and cerebral 'dominance' is necessary to make progress in understanding the fundamentals of the brain code.

In chapter 2, basic topics in neuroanatomy are reviewed. Unlike most neurophysiology texts – with their emphasis on clinical significance or experimental methodology – the emphasis in this chapter is on three structures of importance to higher-level cognition: the cerebral cortex, the so-called 'non-specific' brainstem nuclei, and the corpus callosum, which connects the cortices of the left and right hemispheres.

In chapter 3 clinical and experimental findings and current ideas concerning the corpus callosum are reviewed. A hypothesis concerning the mechanisms of callosal function is presented and illustrated using some elementary computer simulations. Chapter 4 pursues topics related to the psychology of the corpus callosum. Recent findings concerning both the corpus callosum and the high-level cognitive functions of the right hemisphere are reviewed.

Chapter 5 is a brief summary of the main themes of human laterality research and how those themes might be related to the functioning of the corpus callosum. Chapter 6 focuses on several animal experiments which are of direct relevance to the brain code and the involvement of the corpus callosum.

Chapter 7 is a theoretical interlude which places the proposed hypothesis concerning the corpus callosum within the context of general systems theory and the already deciphered codes of nature. Here it is argued that the inhibitory relationship between the cerebral hemispheres is not merely one of many aspects of the functioning of the mammalian brain, but an important part of the brain code.

Finally, chapter 8 is an attempt to tie up loose ends and indicate what implications the callosal hypothesis has for future developments on the brain code and for artificial intelligence in computers.

Throughout the book an attempt has been made to define technical words and phrases as they arise, but a glossary of terms and two appendices are also to be found at the end of the book.

1

INTRODUCTION

The human brain is a mass of interconnecting neurons, the number of which is enormous. Estimates range from 1 to 100 billion neurons, and communications among the neurons are made possible by synapses, the number of which is orders of magnitude larger still. Meanwhile, the computer systems which are used to simulate brain functions contain fewer than 1 million elements and do not show the rich diversity of interconnections which is found in living organisms. This difference in scale between the actual brain and vaguely similar digital computers is so large that many of the mysteries of function, development and ageing of the real brain will undoubtedly remain mysteries for decades to come. Yet, having stated the obvious, it is nonetheless true that a few fundamental characteristics of brain function have been discovered and we can be confident of at least some of the structural pieces and functional relationships which must underlie a realistic theory of brain function. Moreover, such knowledge allows for computer simulations of the activity of small groups of neurons – making possible a second 'experimental' approach, in addition to that involving living brains.

The first insight into brain function was undoubtedly the realization that indeed the brain is the biological organ which allows cognition. Our hearts and livers are important for other reasons, but the brain is the thinker. Secondly, the brain thinks with its massive network of neurons – not its glial cells, blood vessels or cerebrospinal fluid – and the thinking activity of the neurons is fundamentally electrical. The on–off electrical nature of neural activity has led to the familiar computer–brain analogy – the limitations of which we must keep in mind, but there is an important similarity between these two kinds of system: unlike analogies based upon clockwork mechanics or pumps and sluices, the computer analogy is not misleading insofar as neural activity is truly electronic. In detail, there are important differences, but in both cases we are talking about temporal and/or spatial patterns of electrical impulses which allow both systems to compute (see figure 1.1).

Two important facts about brain electronics should be noted. Each neuron is itself a unit which can receive various impulses, 'digest' that input and emit an output. How sophisticated the 'decision-making capabilities' of any one neuron may be remains uncertain, but each neuron is undoubtedly more complex than a small section of copper wire which merely relays all input. Each neuron summates the electrical

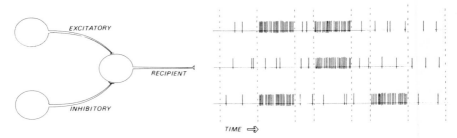

Figure 1.1 Neuronal inhibition and excitation. Here is shown a schematization of the effects of an inhibitory neuron and an excitatory neuron on a third neuron. Increased firing can lead to either a decrease or an increase in the firing of a neuron receiving the axonal output. As far as is now known, no other kinds of 'information' are encoded in the temporal sequence of neuronal firing.

information coming to it both spatially (over the surface of its dendrites, axons and cell body) and temporally (as a serial sequence of such inputs) and responds by exciting or inhibiting other neurons. Secondly, the neuron is unidirectional: the dendrites and axons which, generally speaking, act as the input and output channels to and from the neuronal cell body will normally allow pulses to travel in one direction only. Both of these established facts concerning neuronal function will prove to be important when we consider possible patterns of neural activity in the brain.

The brain code and the neuron code

An essential distinction between the neuron code and the brain code should be noted here. The *neuron code* is the proper subject matter of neuro*physiology* – and that code constitutes the fine-grained substrate of, but is not synonymous with, the *brain code* – which is the proper subject matter of neuro*psychology* in its broadest sense. On the one hand, the neuron code is concerned with the cellular mechanisms by means of which the electrical information in one neuron is summated with that of other neurons and then transmitted to still other neurons. On the other hand, the brain code is concerned with the relatively macroscopic mechanisms by means of which *psychologically meaningful* information (inevitably, multineuron patterns of activity) is transmitted from region to region within the brain.

Although brief discussion of the neuron code will be made in this and the next chapter, the primary concern of psychology and the topic of this book is not in fact the neuron code and the intricacies of cell biology. On the contrary, given certain known mechanisms of neuron-to-neuron communication, we will be interested in considering what kinds of mechanism may be involved as the brain juggles the thoughts and images which we know to be important in normal cognition. For the most part, we will let the cell physiologist worry about which neurotransmitters and how many synapses are involved, and we will concentrate on the relatively macroscopic dynamics of the brain. Again this is a topic for later chapters, but this recurring theme is worth stating clearly at the outset: the results and conclusions of biochemistry, molecular biology and neurophysiology will necessarily provide most of the bricks and mortar of a theory of the brain, but such building blocks are neither equivalent to nor do they add up simply and obviously to the neuronal cathedral which we are trying to understand. Provided with a firm grasp of the well-established aspects of neuron science, still our work in unraveling the puzzle of the brain has just begun.

Fortunately the bricks-and-mortar science of the brain has advanced remarkably over the past three decades. Most importantly, it has become possible to record the electrical activity of single cells in the living brain. Such single-cell recording experiments have shown un-equivocally that one important aspect of the neuron code is simple firing rate. A given neuron in primary visual cortex, for example, will fire more frequently when a visual stimulus has certain (location, intensity, wave-length and/or orientation) characteristics, and less frequently when one or more of the relevant features of the stimulus are changed.

As yet little is known about the significance of the actual temporal sequence of the firing of a particular cell (or the significance of the interburst interval and other higher-order temporal features of the firing series). Especially as sensory information in various modalities is mixed together in association cortex, it may well be that more complex temporal codes related to the probabilities of simultaneous stimuli play an important role in abstracting high-level information from the sensory field. For example, the pattern of visual information which at some region of visual cortex is translated into the concept of 'dog' may be decoded as a neutral stimulus unless associated with the sounds of a dog barking. Depending upon the frequency with which this combina-tion of stimuli has been associated with physical pain or other types of distress, these independently neutral stimuli may take on new mean-ings. In this example, it is the simultaneity of the auditory and visual stimuli which signals the potential danger.

In other words, the temporal sequence of neuronal firing is likely to be an important aspect of the *neuron* code in abstracting information from sensory stimuli, but it is noteworthy that the information ab-stracted from a temporal sequence is itself likely to be stored topographi-cally (that is, spatially) on the cortex. The simplest manifestation of this process of translating the temporal dimension into spatial dimen-sions is the localization of high-frequency sounds anteriorly within primary auditory cortex, with lower frequencies located posteriorly. The actual firing rate of the cortical neurons involved does not affect the frequency of the perceived tone. Such 'spatialization' of the temporal dimension in the cortex is arguably one of the primary functions of the *neuron* code.

The detailed mechanisms involved in the neuron code will un-doubtedly continue to fascinate the cell physiologist for decades to come, but the implications for the psychologist lie primarily in the fact that, however the brain code may work, it works in a world which is greatly simplified in terms of its temporal characteristics. The extremely high frequencies of photic stimulation, the lower frequencies of audi-tory stimulation and the extremely low frequencies of tactile stimula-tion are all translated into an artificial two-dimensional world where the on or off signals of neurons individually 'mean' stimulation of peripheral sense organs at a given frequency quite unrelated to the frequency of the cortical neuron firing.

The relationship between temporal and spatial encoding of sensory stimuli will be explored in later chapters. Suffice it to say that there are mechanisms for both temporal and spatial summation in the brain – some of which appear to be like the high-speed serial computations of computers and some of which appear to be like the topographical encoding of environmental stimuli on to a suitably sensitive 'neuronal photographic film.'

Progress in determining the precise computational and sensory map-ping mechanisms of the brain continues to be rapid. Currently several lacunae in our understanding of the cell physiology of the *neuron code* remain, but need not imply that elucidation of the fundamentals of the *brain code* will be impossible. Today we can be sure of the importance of at least two temporal aspects of the neuron code: the more frequent the firing of a given neuron, the more frequent *or* the less frequent the firing of those neurons receiving its axonal output. In other words, we can be sure of only excitatory and inhibitory relationships among neurons – the degree of the effect being a function of the firing rate. More complex things may in fact be happening between neurons, but we will see that already excitation/inhibition – unrelated to complex temporal factors – has direct implications for the brain code.

Evolution of the brain – the 'vertical' dimension

Climbing up the 'tree' of animal evolution, it is apparent that there are massive increases in the number of, and complexity of connections among, the neurons in animal brains. This is generally true in terms of the absolute numbers of neurons and is particularly striking in terms of the number of neurons relative to various measures of body size. But the essence of this increase in size and complexity is better understood in terms of the amount of nervous tissue interposed between nerve fibers carrying sensory input from the body surface and nerve fibers carrying motor output to effector organs. One such measure is the ratio of the size of the cerebral cortex relative to the number of ascending and descending nerve fibers – a better indicator than brain volume of the degree of brain activity intervening between stimulus and response. Thinking along these lines, various attempts at devising objective anatomical measures of the spectrum of animal intelligence have been made within the field of comparative neuroanatomy.

The underlying hope has been that if evolutionary changes in brain structure can be related to behavioral differences among species, then some progress in understanding how the brain thinks will be possible. It is surprising, however, how difficult it has proven to obtain a simple measure of the brain which reflects the phylogenetic development of a species – much less a measure which reflects intelligence or specific behaviors.

Absolute brain size (table 1.1) suggests a strong correlation between greater intelligence (or complexity of behavior) and absolute body weight, whereas this is apparently not the case either within a species or across species. Big animals are not necessarily smart ones.

Table 1.1   Brain sizes (in grams)

1	whale	6,800	29	mangabey	98
2	elephant	4,717	30	macacus melanotus	80
3	dolphin	1,735	31	rhesus monkey	80
4	man	1,444	32	dog	79
5	walrus	1,126	33	macacus sinus	67
6	camel	762	34	fox	53
7	giraffe	680	35	porcupine	38
8	hippopotamus	582	36	domestic cat	25
9	horse	532	37	crocodile	16
10	polar bear	498	38	alligator	14
11	ox	493	39	rabbit	9
12	chimpanzee	440	40	marmoset	7
13	deer	411	41	common squirrel	6.1
14	donkey	385	42	guinea pig	4.7
15	orang-utan	372	43	brown rat	2.4
16	seal	271	44	flying squirrel	1.9
17	antelope	269	45	iguana	1.4
18	tiger	263	46	vampire bat	1.2
19	monitor	244	47	gila monster	0.73
20	lion	241	48	house mouse	0.43
21	grizzly bear	234	49	water vole	0.36
22	wild pig	178	50	tortoise	0.30
23	sheep	140	51	black snake	0.29
24	baboon	137	52	bull frog	0.24
25	wolf	119	53	lizard	0.12
26	domestic pig	113	54	common viper	0.11
27	macaque monkey	106	55	common frog	0.09
28	gibbon	102	56	common toad	0.07

Source: data from table 128 of Blinkov and Glezer (1968).

To eliminate the body-size factor, the ratio of brain size to body size has been examined, but conversely this index unduly favors various small animals (table 1.2) – with the flying squirrel and the devastatingly brilliant monitor finishing higher on this scale of intelligence than *Homo sapiens*. As seen in these tables, the spectrum of intelligence suggested by absolute brain weight may please those of us with a special dislike of snakes and frogs – and that suggested by brain/body ratios may offer some solace to those of us with a special fear of alligators, but neither measure gives man and the other primates their proper distinction.

The counter-intuitive nature of the hierarchies of intelligence in tables 1.1 and 1.2 has led to more complex coefficients of intelligence which are applicable only within specific limited groups (primates, mammals, etc.) (see Jerison, 1973, for a detailed discussion). From an evolutionary perspective, there are indeed grounds for arguing that rigorous comparisons will be possible only within such 'lines' of related

Table 1.2 Brain weight/Body weight ratios

1	macacus melanotus	1:14	29	wild pig	1:315
2	mangabey	1:14	30	common frog	1:383
3	macacus sinus	1:14	31	sheep	1:393
4	baboon	1:18	32	porcupine	1:400
5	rhesus monkey	1:20	33	lizard	1:413
6	marmoset	1:29	34	donkey	1:455
7	monitor	1:31	35	polar bear	1:519
8	flying squirrel	1:33	36	camel	1:525
9	antelope	1:37	37	walrus	1:592
10	man	1:44	38	common toad	1:610
11	seal	1:47	39	grizzly bear	1:611
12	house mouse	1:48	40	common viper	1:611
13	common squirrel	1:53	41	lion	1:626
14	gibbon	1:60	42	elephant	1:646
15	vampire bat	1:77	43	horse	1:692
16	macaque monkey	1:82	44	tiger	1:700
17	dolphin	1:82	45	gila monster	1:704
18	fox	1:87	46	giraffe	1:778
19	chimpanzee	1:128	47	whale	1:854
20	domestic cat	1:129	48	bull frog	1:1,002
21	rabbit	1:132	49	tortoise	1:1,067
22	guinea pig	1:148	50	domestic pig	1:1,327
23	dog	1:170	51	ox	1:1,339
24	brown rat	1:190	52	black snake	1:1,481
25	wolf	1:191	53	iguana	1:2,910
26	orang-utan	1:196	54	hippopotamus	1:3,015
27	water vole	1:254	55	crocodile	1:8,590
28	deer	1:305	56	alligator	1:12,976

Source: data from table 128 of Blinkov and Glezer (1968).

organisms – and quantitative methods in comparative neuroanatomy currently focus on such subgroups. Yet without arguing against such techniques, it is nonetheless true that they cannot answer some of the questions which originally motivated research in comparative neuroanatomy. If we study evolutionary subgroups separately, how can we obtain an answer to questions about the relative intelligence of man, the dolphin and the songbirds? And can any conclusions be drawn about the human brain from assorted findings from comparative anatomy, such as the fact that the electric eel has a relatively large cerebellum or that the lion has a large amygdala?

The relative intelligence of animal species may seem a prize topic for setting academics to sleep in their armchairs, but it is a part of a larger question of obvious importance. If behavior is controlled by (or at least through) the brain, then behavioral differences should reflect (or be reflected in) differences in brain function. When we are angry or fearful or attentive or confused, there simply must be characteristic brain states which are as consistent and replicable as are such cognitive states.

In the final analysis a complete 'brain code' would delineate what those differences are. At a more academic level we should be able to determine what, for example, the major neuronal differences are between the domestic dog and the wild wolf. Structurally their brains are very similar, but somewhere there are anatomical/physiological distinctions which make the dog amenable to domestic life and the wolf almost never so. What furthermore distinguishes the brains of schizophrenics from the brains of people capable of more or less normal social existence? Clearly we are yet a long way from explaining species differences, much less personality differences or psychiatric states in terms of brain structures, so that most research efforts have remained at the preliminary level of trying to correlate the crudest measures of personality, behavior or intelligence with the grossest measures of the brain itself.

In the study of animal species the ratio of cortical surface area to bulbar cross-section (a measure of the number of fibers ascending and descending through the brainstem) gets us closer to the expected hierarchy of intelligence, because we are then evaluating the degree of 'excess' brain matter beyond that needed for sensation and motor control of the body. The deficiency of this scale is that there is still a bias in favor of small animals. Ideally we would like to find a biological measure which is not affected by the size of the animal and which is applicable to a wide range of species.

Unfortunately no such measure has become established, but an interesting start has been made in Anthony's (1938) 'calloso-bulbar ratio'. As shown in figure 1.2, the calloso-bulbar ratio reflects the amount of nervous tissue devoted to communication between the left and right cerebral hemispheres, relative to the amount of tissue devoted to receiving/sending impulses up and down the spinal cord. Strictly

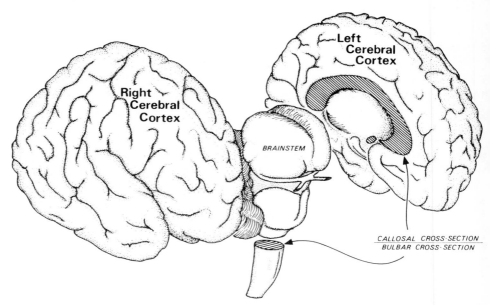

Figure 1.2 A particularly good index of brain evolution. The 'calloso-bulbar ratio,' illustrated in this figure, is a measure of the amount of hemispheric cross-talk relative to the amount of information flowing through the brainstem. Both the vertical and horizontal values are obtained merely as cross-sectional measures, and are therefore only rough estimates of the amount of interhemispheric communication insofar as differences in the diameters of individual nerve fibers are ignored.

speaking such an index is appropriate only for animals with a corpus callosum – excluding the marsupials (kangaroos, etc.), the songbirds and all reptiles, and so on – but a comparable index could be developed simply in terms of the number of forebrain commissural fibers joining the cerebral hemispheres. A 'commissuro-bulbar index' – being the ratio of commissural fibers (above the brainstem) divided by the number of ascending and descending brainstem fibers – would not exclude the marsupials, the lower vertebrates or the songbirds and therefore would allow comparison among diverse species (see table 1.3).

Three definitions of important brain structures which are shown in figure 1.2 should be noted. The *cerebral cortex* is the outer 2–3 mm of the entire surface of the cerebral hemispheres. Since the cell bodies of neurons lie here, the total area of the cortex has often been thought of as a rough measure of animal intelligence. Below the cortex is the subcortex, which is the mass of input and output fibers to and from the cortex. Its size is directly related to the size of the cortex. Below the subcortex (and several nuclei imbedded within it) lies the centrally located *brainstem*. Although most tracts and nuclei within the brainstem also come in bilateral pairs, their anatomical separateness is less clear than that of the cerebral hemispheres, and there are relatively far

Table 1.3 Calloso-bulbar index

Species	Index
Man	3.12
Chimpanzee	1.79
Baboon	1.39
Guenon	1.19
Elephant	1.11
Brown bear	1.07
Polar bear	1.06
Dolphin	0.93
Wolf	0.89
Horse	0.70
Lion	0.67
Fox	0.62
Hippopotamus	0.56
Lemur	0.32

Source: from table 179 of Blinkov and Glezer (1968).

more commissural fibers joining both sides. Within the brainstem lies most of the control centers regulating the so-called autonomic nervous system. Finally the term, *commissures*, refers to all fibers which cross the midline to connect the left and right sides of the central nervous system. The so-called forebrain commissures are all such fibers which are found above the level of the brainstem. In the human brain (and many mammals) more than 90 percent of all the forebrain commissural fibers are contained within the *corpus callosum*. For most purposes, therefore, it is sufficient to discuss only the corpus callosum when considering the nature of the communication between the left and right cerebral cortices.

It would of course be difficult and of dubious value to ascertain the relative intelligence of the hippopotamus and the polar bear, but it may be significant that a brain measure which puts *Homo sapiens* at the top with the chimpanzee finishing a poor second is one which takes into account a measure of the amount of cerebral hemispheric cross-talk. In other words, even for an understanding of the major trends in brain evolution, it may not be enough to speak only of the 'vertical' growth of the nervous system. (And in chapter 4 we will see that interhemispheric communication is in fact important for certain aspects of normal human intelligence.)

Bilateral symmetry – the 'horizontal' dimension

An alien from outer space would probably soon discover the phylogenetic scale on earth and make contact with the dolphin, songbirds and various primates. But even before attempting to make sense of the significance of brain size (relative to body weight, or cortical area, or some less obvious measure of the beast), the alien would undoubtedly need to satisfy its curiosity about the bilateral symmetry of the vast majority of creatures in the animal kingdom. Almost wherever it looked, the alien would find the local inhabitants to be mirror-images of themselves joined at the vertical midline.

The why of bilateral symmetry can perhaps be answered in terms of the advantages conferred by such symmetry for locomotion in both aquatic and terrestrial environments. Early in evolution bilaterally constructed nervous systems may have allowed primitive organisms to get around more efficiently than their rotating or spiraling friends – and the pressures of natural selection would have subsequently led to a diversity of descendants who wriggle, strut or swim left, then right, then left.

But the implications of bilateral symmetry in higher organisms are both more complex and fortunately more interesting. In an organism with two roughly similar 'brains,' the two halves must in some way coordinate their activities to allow for the successful locomotion of the organism as a whole. This cooperation between the left and right may take various forms, but the anatomical separateness of the cerebral hemispheres must not lead us glibly to conclusions about their independence. It is their *cooperation* which allows us to walk – presumably mutual inhibition which lets one foot go forward while the other remains behind. And it may be mutual excitation which allows the kangaroo to hop and birds to fly. Whatever the detailed mechanism that is involved, clearly *independence* would be disastrous. In other words, despite the anatomical separateness of the left and right cerebral hemispheres, a major concern in trying to understand how the nervous system works should be to understand how the two halves work together.

The nature of the cooperation between the cerebral hemispheres of bilaterally symmetrical nervous systems will concern us throughout this book, but it should be clear that this is *not* an esoteric footnote in neurology. Not only is it an anatomical fact that all bilaterally symmetrical nervous systems have extensive connections across the midline at all levels, but also two further facts from neuroanatomy indicate that this is an extremely important feature of the human nervous system: (i) the *largest* single nerve tract in the human nervous system is one such commissure – the corpus callosum, which connects the cortices of the two cerebral hemispheres, and (ii) the corpus callosum is the *fastest* growing tract in evolution. In other words, whatever kinds of hemispheric interactions are allowed by the corpus callosum, their importance – as judged by the amount of nervous tissue devoted to their functions – is increasing in evolution and increasing more rapidly than even the growth in the total area of the cerebral cortex.

If in fact the major themes of the evolution of the animal brain include both increases in neocortical area *and* increases in the number of fibers connecting the left and right cortices to one another, then it may well be that an understanding of the workings of the human brain depends crucially on understanding both the mechanisms of cortical information storage *and* the mechanisms by which two such memory banks communicate (the functions of the corpus callosum).

First steps toward the brain code

In the roughest terms we know that both the horizontal and the vertical aspects of brain organization must be included in our description of the brain code, but it is far from obvious how to proceed from such general, macroscopic considerations. We can easily surmise that, when we discuss the flow of information in the brain, we must consider both the flow *within* each hemisphere and the flow *between* the hemispheres. But how can these two processes be related to each other? The theoretical framework which has guided my own thinking in this area is outlined in chapter 7, but it may be instructive at this point to consider briefly those codes of nature which have already been deciphered.

The 'genetic code' of cell biology describes the flow of information among the macromolecules found in living cells. That code was deciphered in a relatively short period following the elucidation of the structure of DNA by Watson and Crick in 1953. Once the helical configuration of the DNA – with its sugar and phosphate backbone and the inward orientation of the nucleotide bases – became known, the number of ways in which the purine and pyrimidines could be aligned was severely limited and the mechanism of gene replication soon became evident. Moreover once the principle of nucleotide base-pairing had become known, an understanding of the processes of RNA transcription and of translation to amino acid sequences was not far off. In fact Crick had already theoretically worked out the major features of the translation process by 1958, several years prior to explicit empirical verification of this portion of the genetic code.

In atomic physics attainment of a fundamental understanding of the 'atomic code' also awaited the discovery of a relatively small number of crucial structural facts concerning the atom and its nucleus. Nineteenth-century chemistry had indeed revealed some periodic features of the known elements, but not until the reality of the nucleus had been established did the quantal structure of the nucleus's electron cover and the meaning of chemical valence became clear. And not until the discovery of the neutron by Chadwick in 1931 did the quantal structure of the nucleus and its nuclear periodicities begin to be understood.

It is now known that the principal information exchanges within living cells are well described by the 'central dogma' of molecular biology:

$$DNA \longleftrightarrow RNA \rightarrow Protein$$

And atomic physics has a comparable if less frequently noted 'central dogma:'

$$Neutron \longleftrightarrow Proton \rightarrow Electron$$

Each 'dogma' indicates those interactions which are important for the functioning of the given system and, by omission, those interactions which do not occur or are, in some way, unimportant. Due principally to the establishment of these conceptual frameworks, in terms of which virtually all known aspects of the cell and the atom can now be

Table 1.4 Atomic and cellular research as classified in relation to the central dogmas of atomic physics and molecular biology

1	4	2	5	3
Neutron	⇄	Proton	⇄	Electron
	6		7	

1 neutron–neutron interactions: the 'pure' nuclear force.
2 proton–proton interactions: the Coulomb force at large distances, the Coulomb and nuclear forces at small distances (nuclear fission, fusion, radioactive decay).
3 electron–electron interactions: the Coulomb force, van der Waals forces, hydrophobic–hydrophilic interactions.
4, 6 neutron–proton interactions: the nuclear force.
5 proton effects on electrons: the Coulomb force, much of organic and inorganic chemistry and solid-state physics.
7 electron effects on protons: the Coulomb force, electron effects on nuclear structure and fission rates.

1	4	2	5	3
DNA	⇄	RNA	⇄	Protein
	6		7	

1 DNA replication: molecular genetics.
2 RNA replication: virus research.
3 protein–protein interactions: protein affinity studies.
4 transcription: cell differentiation studies, etc.
5 translation: cell differentiation studies, etc.
6 reverse transcription: virus research, cancer research, cell differentiation studies, etc.
7 reverse translation: unknown. [1]

Note: 1. See Mekler (1967); Cook (1977, 1980b); Wassermann (1982, 1983).

understood, both molecular biology and atomic physics have entered stages of mature development (see table 1.4).

At higher levels of natural organization, there is yet very little known about the fundamental information 'codes' by which more complex systems run. Certainly within psychology there is no single accepted paradigm around which most research is organized and no 'central dogma' concerning which agreement has been reached. Although it is well established that the neuron is the fundamental functional unit of the brain and that inhibitory and excitatory relationships among neurons are fundamental processes, those indisputable facts have led perhaps neurophysiology, but certainly not psychology, into a stage of mature growth.

Without a central paradigm to guide the search for physiological and psychological correlates, psychology has remained in a 'post-Mendelian/pre-DNA' stage of development (or perhaps a 'post-periodic chart/pre-quantum theory' stage). In other words, systematic regularities in both physiological and psychological data have been discovered, but there is still no core theory to bind the two realms together. It is as though psychologists were collecting data in the manner of the pre-modern chemists – some classifying their substances by color, some by odor, some by boiling point – and with each system proving itself to be self-consistent in its own way. But none of these 'modern' psychological systems maps unambiguously on to a second system, while each system is proclaimed by its proponents to be *the* fundamental perspective around which all branches of psychology eventually must be built.

Having said this, I do not believe that the psychologist needs to be apologetic. The subject matter of psychology – even if restricted to human/animal behavior and excluding perennial problems concerning the nature of mind and consciousness – is orders of magnitude more complex than the subject matters of atomic physics and cellular biology. Being constructed of atoms and cells, it is unlikely that animal organisms and their behavior would be *less* complex than their components. It is not therefore unreasonable to expect that the fundamentals of animal behavior would be understood only subsequent to the attainment of an understanding of those constituent pieces.

Moreover the time-scale of major developments in atomic physics and cellular biology suggests that the deciphering of the brain code is yet a few years away. In atomic physics the nature of atomic organization became known subsequent to: (i) the discovery of the electron by Thompson (1897), (ii) the discovery of the nucleus by Rutherford (1911), (iii) the discovery of the neutron by Chadwick (1931), and (iv) the formulation of the laws of quantum mechanics (1900–32). In cellular biology the major themes of cellular organization became known subsequent to: (i) the discovery of the genetic importance of the nucleic acids (1935), (ii) the discovery that DNA is the genetic material by Avery (1944), (iii) the elucidation of the structure of DNA by Watson and Crick (1953), (iv) the discovery of the translation process by Jacob and Monod (1963), and (v) the rediscovery and formalization of the laws of Mendelian inheritance (1900–40). Assuming that the fundamental themes of atomic structure became understood over the three decades prior to 1932 and those of the cell over the three decades prior to 1963, perhaps we are not being too lenient in giving the psychologist a 1994 deadline for cracking the brain code!

Be that as it may, as of today a 'central dogma' in psychology has not been promulgated, but the utter simplicity of the central dogmas which brought order to atomic physics and molecular biology is well worth noting. Essentially three elements plus their allowed and disallowed interactions are all that they are comprised of. Behind this simplicity of control mechanisms, there of course lies all the complexities of quantum physics and the biology of living forms – but the core concepts in these realms are succinct and unambiguous (table 1.4).

Perhaps therefore we can expect similar simplicity in the psychological realm, but it must be said that we do not know for certain whether or not the fundamental materials from which to build a psychological 'central dogma' have in fact been discovered. Prior to the discovery of the electron or prior to the characterization of DNA as a sequence of nucleotide bases, it would have been madness to talk about any hint of 'dogma' at those levels of organization. If it is today the case that in psychology we still lack truly fundamental facts concerning brain function, then all attempts at describing 'the brain code' would be doomed from the start. Yet within the abundance of empirical findings in neuroscience, it is entirely possible that the building blocks of a 'central dogma' for psychology have in fact been discovered, but not yet seen to be fundamental. In other words, our inability to propound a 'central dogma' may be more a conceptual problem than an experimental one. Unfortunately there is no way of demonstrating from abstract arguments whether we have or have not collected the necessary building materials, and so we must proceed by constructing some hypotheses to see if they hold together and lead in fruitful directions.

As our first steps towards the brain code, let us first of all ask two of the nagging questions which continue to haunt human neuropsychology – the answers to which will undoubtedly contribute to our understanding of the brain code.

WHY IS THERE BILATERAL *ASYMMETRY* OF FUNCTION IN THE HUMAN BRAIN?

If we and most other animal species have roughly bilaterally symmetrical nervous systems, why do nearly all people have a favored hand for writing and other skilled manipulations of the external world and why is the ability to generate speech limited to one hemisphere?

Some very clever arguments have been devised to answer these questions based upon the left-handed twisting of the DNA molecule, the off-center position of the heart, the asymmetric nature of human egg cells at the time of fertilization, and so on. Those hypotheses concerned with fundamental asymmetries in nature may indeed have a place in the final explanation of hemispheric asymmetries, but on their own they suffer from overprediction. Certainly if we were to argue that something as ubiquitous as the molecular asymmetry of DNA somehow biases all living creatures to the left then such a theory would predict more extensive asymmetries of animal nervous systems than the occasional oversized crab claw and left-sided speech dominance in man!

Given the directionality of the DNA helix and the known asymmetries of racemic compounds, etc. there may very well be a pervasive asymmetrical structural bias throughout the natural world. All things being equal, a microscopic asymmetry might become manifest in macroscopic, organismic asymmetries, but we must not lose sight of the primary facts which have led psychologists to consider this question of asymmetries in nature. Above and beyond all the many other intriguing asymmetric curiosities, that which needs explaining is why speech capabilities are found in only one – not both – hemispheres in 95 percent of the normal human population and why some 90 percent of this majority of people generate speech from the left side of the brain. Next we must be able to account for handedness – with again a strong bias for left-hemispheric dominance. In explaining these two well-established facts, we must also be able to provide a plausible argument to account for why so *few* other species share our apparent need for cerebral asymmetry of function. Only when we have put these major issues within a sensible theoretical framework will it be worthwhile to explore the miniscule differences in the processing of musical melodies, facial expressions and other talents often said to have a favored side in the brain.

Although unanimity of opinion may not have been reached, one predominant view among psychologists is that the most fundamental cerebral asymmetry may be a *motor* asymmetry for the control of *speech*. Certainly on theoretical grounds, the advantages of unilateral 'dominance' appear to be most straightforward in terms of speech capabilities. The hands and both feet have their primary neural control centers in the contralateral hemisphere and should therefore work somewhat independently – not unlike the independence between our arms and legs as we run and swing a tennis racket and between our legs and speech organs as we walk and talk. It is therefore not obvious from first principles why one hand or one foot would be functionally more competent than its partner. Unlike the skilled use of the hand or foot, however, speech is neurologically a somewhat unusual motor event because the *midline* organs of speech – the lips, tongue, throat and vocal cords – are innervated equally from both sides. There is consequently a far greater potential for hemispheric conflict, interference and disagreements in the control of organs located on the midline of the body than on the far periphery where there is at least a strong predominance of neural control from the contralateral hemisphere. Control of speech by only one hemisphere may be a simple means of avoiding confusion.

In other words (and as Jones, 1966, Moscovitch, 1973, Sperry, 1974, Passingham, 1981, and Stein, 1983, have argued previously), there is a reasonable theoretical argument for expecting unilateral dominance for overt speech activities – simply to allow for unambiguous control of midline organs. Conversely unambiguous and consistent unilateral hemispheric dominance would *not* arise in any species which does not require fine motor control of midline organs. That is nearly all non-human species, with the notable exception of the songbirds, would *not* show functional asymmetry. The issue of cerebral dominance in species other than man will be discussed in more detail in chapter 6, but it is noteworthy that clear cerebral dominance has been demonstrated only in certain species of songbird – with again left-sided dominance in the songbird's means of social communication (Nottebohm, 1977).

The argument that cerebral dominance may be a direct consequence of unilateral motor control of speech (and communicative birdsong) has been presented in greater detail and more eloquently by others (see Stein, 1983). Although why both man and the songbirds show unilateral dominance on the *left* side of the brain is not answered in this hypothesis, it does reduce much of the laterality literature to one central argument – with admittedly some loose ends yet to be taken care of. In this view, (i) one hemisphere emerged dominant for the control of midline organs (during speech) to prevent hemispheric conflict; (ii) dominance for speech *production* led inextricably to dominance for speech *comprehension* (the 'motor hypothesis of speech perception' (Liberman *et al.*, 1967)); and (iii) this unilateral capability freed the right hemisphere for other kinds of 'dominance.' Point (iii) remains the least clear in this view of lateral dominance – primarily because the mentioned need for speech dominance does not indicate what kinds of non-speech activity the 'non-dominant' hemisphere might be engaged in. Specifically what does it mean to say that the right hemisphere is 'freed' for other kinds of specializations?

WHAT IS THE RIGHT HEMISPHERE DOING?

So let us tentatively accept this argument concerning the speech dominance of the left hemisphere and even tag on a few corollary arguments. Let us say that the use of midline organs requires unilateral dominance, and further that this motor dominance allows the left hemisphere to become more efficient at both encoding *and* decoding the phonetic elements of language. Therefore despite the nearly complete bilateral symmetry of all sensory stimulation, the involvement of motor activity in speech comprehension gives one hemisphere (usually the left) both a motor and a sensory advantage over its otherwise perfectly competent partner on the right. Furthermore let us assume a small tendency for this motor superiority to spill over to a handedness and 'footedness' advantage related to the same hemisphere. Having established itself as the expressive 'executive,' the speech-dominant hemisphere then has a slight tendency to become the executive in other skilled actions – primarily those involving the use of one hand. In other words, let us pretend for the moment that we have in fact explained the major features of unilateral cerebral motor *dominance*. Still we are left with a difficult question: What is the right hemisphere doing while the left hemisphere is busy with the chores of linguistic communication?

As will become clear in chapter 4, I believe that this is one of the most important *unanswered* questions in neuropsychology. Some would undoubtedly assert that it has already been adequately answered: whereas the left hemisphere manipulates words, the right hemisphere manipulates visual images (or emotions, or melodies, etc.). And I would acknowledge that there is some truth to this multifarious lateralized specializations view of cerebral dominance. Yet serious consideration of the nature of hemispheric interactions via the forebrain commissures demands that we ask what one hemisphere is doing *simultaneously* with the 'dominant' functions of the other hemisphere. If the cerebral hemispheres are indeed as 'yoked' to one another as the massive commissural connections suggest, then the activity on one side must somehow result in complementary activity (in an unknown, but physiologically precise way) on the other side. Furthermore if the cerebral hemispheres act *together* under virtually all normal conditions – receiving nearly identical sensory stimuli and at least not competing during most motor output, then suggestions of pairs of 'hemispheric talents' are not helpful for an understanding of brain function, *unless a functional relationship can be demonstrated between them*. Marshall (1981) has made a similar complaint in this way: 'Descriptive dichotomies (either absolute or relative) pose rather than answer the question of what distinguishes the hemispheres.'

As an example of an unhelpful dichotomy, consider the 'verbal-visuospatial' characterization of the cerebral hemispheres. In this view, a normal conversation between two people could be described as verbal exchanges between the respective left hemispheres – while the right hemispheres detect the changes in facial expression, body posture, 'meaningful glances,' etc., of the other individual. Again this characterization of brain functions may contain some grains of truth, but it presents two major – and I believe insurmountable – problems. First of all, there is an immense imbalance in the informational load of the two hemispheres implied in this view. The left hemisphere is seen as dealing with the entire realm of abstract conceptual thought and the right hemisphere is virtually locked into its sensory field. Only Eccles (1977) appears to have fully appreciated this gross imbalance, but instead of concluding that such a dichotomy is therefore unlikely to be correct, he accepts it and takes it to its logical – and I believe incorrect –

conclusion. In his view only the left hemisphere is characteristically 'human' and 'conscious,' while the right hemisphere is 'instinctual' and 'unconscious.' But the assertion that two neural structures as similar as the cerebral hemispheres could have such qualitatively different functions is, at best, implausible and, at worst, requires invocation of metaphysical arguments to explain how one hemisphere is conscious and the other is unconscious.

Secondly, even if we were to try to elevate the right hemisphere to the status of an equal partner – involved, for example, in the 'affective' components of thought processes – there is no obvious link between the functions on one side and those on the other: promulgation of a dichotomy does not establish the necessary dynamic relationship. Instead of the 'two cooperating halves' of the brain, such views inevitably lead to ideas about 'two brains' or 'two selves': the left 'self' spending most of its time and energy in frontal and parietal association cortex, while the right 'self' enjoys the pleasures of visual cortex and the thrills of the right half of the limbic system! Caricature, to be sure, but how can the 'separate specializations' view of the cerebral hemispheres avoid such unlikely gross asymmetries?

While we cannot be content with suggestions of functional dichotomies which imply a gross imbalance in the informational content of the cerebral hemispheres and which provide no reasonable organic relationship between the functions, the dual anatomical nature of the cerebral hemispheres invites – perhaps demands – suggestions of func-

Table 1.5 Dichotomies attributed to the cerebral hemispheres

Left hemisphere	Right hemisphere
Experimentally derived	
sequential	parallel or simultaneous
analytic	synthetic
linguistic	visuospatial
verbal	nonverbal
focal	diffuse
local	global
linear	spatial
mathematical	geometric
Philosophically motivated	
expressive	perceptive
propositional	appositional
symbolic	imaginative
intellection	emotion
reason	affect
discrete	holistic
active	passive
logical	intuitive

tional dichotomies. Many such dichotomies have been proposed (table 1.5), but few have survived as more than convenient shorthand half-truths!

The first such dichotomy – the verbal/nonverbal characterization – was derived from clinical studies of brain-damaged patients. A strong tendency was found for language functions to be disrupted when the left hemisphere was damaged, whereas right-sided damage had various, but less easily characterized, and much less debilitating effects. Indeed, so striking were the deficits which were produced in a small number of such patients in the mid-1800s that the related brain areas were labeled after the astute physicians involved (figure 1.3). 'Broca's area' is a small portion of the left frontal lobe, damage to which characteristically results in difficulties in speech production, while language comprehension remains intact. Conversely 'Wernicke's area' is a portion of the temporo-parietal region, damage to which affects language comprehension, but not production.

Speculations concerning right-hemisphere functions also date from the middle of the nineteenth century when J. H. Jackson suggested that an 'expression/perception' cognitive dichotomy is embodied in the left and right cerebral hemispheres. By 'perception' Jackson meant high-level comprehension (including the comprehension of language), as distinct from mere 'sensation.' This dichotomy was apparently based upon little more than the suspicion that, although mute, the other half of the brain is likely to be involved in high-level cognition which is in some way complementary to the expressive capabilities of the dominant hemisphere. A similar high-level role of the right hemisphere was later

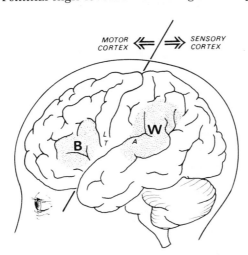

Figure 1.3 The left hemisphere. The two major speech 'centers.' Broca's area (B), located just anterior from the cortical regions for motor control of the lips (L) and tongue (T), and Wernicke's area (W), located at the junction of auditory, visual and somatosensory cortical areas – posterior from the primary auditory cortex (A).

advocated by Penfield (1959), who suggested that it contains a 'conceptual mechanism' which is complementary to the 'speech mechanisms' on the left.

Unfortunately the inability to pin-point and manipulate experimentally right-hemisphere functions led ultimately to the widespread acceptance of a 'dominant/non-dominant' characterization – the right hemisphere being viewed most easily in terms of what it isn't. It might be argued that the 'non-dominant' description of the right hemisphere was for many years the safest label for this unknown entity on the right, but instead of implying 'unknown,' it came to imply 'inferior' and 'subordinate,' and, as such, the non-language hemisphere and non-linguistic cognitive skills were grossly underestimated for nearly a century.

Starting in 1949 unilateral injection of an anesthetic drug into the left or right carotid artery leading toward the brain (the Wada test) was used by neurosurgeons to produce brief disruption of the functions of one hemisphere at a time – a technique useful for determining the 'language hemisphere.' Although some interesting findings concerning the emotional reactivity of each side have been reported, the rapid recovery from the effects of the drug prevents detailed testing of right-hemisphere capabilities. Only the most obvious behavioral deficits can be observed during the two or three minutes of anesthesia. Again the one unambiguous finding using this technique concerns the localization of expressive speech: most patients stop talking after left-sided injection, but not after right-sided injection – thus supporting the verbal/non-verbal dichotomy.

Modern clinical work and non-invasive techniques in normal subjects have continued to support the 'speech/something else' dichotomy, but not until the beginning of the so-called 'split-brain' research did it become possible to investigate directly what the isolated right hemisphere can do. As a last resort treatment, the corpus callosum (and sometimes other forebrain commissures) has been transected in a small number of epilepsy patients. Although they have inevitably had a long history of severe epileptic seizures, some of them show no gross abnormalities of brain structures, so their separated cerebral hemispheres have been studied – with fingers crossed – as representative of normal hemispheric functions. The most unambiguous, but not by any means the only finding concerning right-hemisphere talents has been in the realm of visuospatial perception and manipulation. When asked to draw a picture, identify complex shapes, work through mazes or otherwise perform tasks in a complex two- or three-dimensional space, the right hemisphere outperforms the previously presumed 'dominant' left hemisphere (Gazzaniga, 1970). Therefore the first myth to fall in the light of modern split-brain research was the dominant/nondominant dichotomy. Hemispheric 'dominance' apparently depends on the task at hand, although the 'dominance' of the right hemisphere is not usually evident in normal subjects due to the habitual use of language in interacting with the external world.

The techniques used on these patients have been borrowed and refined for use in normal subjects and a host of functional dichotomies have been suggested (table 1.5). The empirical basis for some of these dichotomies will be discussed in later chapters.

The dichotomies inferred from empirical studies often lack the 'balance' and psychological profundity which are contained in the dichotomies offered from philosophical viewpoints (table 1.5), but something of a common thread seems to have emerged. The left hemisphere is said to be more precise, more analytic, more linear and more literal in its perception and manipulation of the outside world. The right hemisphere is said to be more diffuse, more holistic, more geometric and more involved with the 'overall picture' when it is called upon. But can we find some physiological mechanisms which will imply psychological dichotomies of this kind?

Summary

The 'vertical dimension' of the brain can be succinctly summarized in terms of the evolutionary trends in brain structure. The brains of the lower vertebrates show little development of association areas – limited to the associational capacities of the limbic system, whereas mammalian and particularly primate brains show massive increases in neocortical tissue interposed between sensory input and motor output. In a word, the higher vertebrates have a much greater neural capacity to manipulate and evaluate sensory information prior to emitting a behavioral response.

The 'horizontal dimension' of brain organization has shown very little change in evolution in the sense that approximate bilateral symmetry has remained the general rule, but at least two evolutionary trends can also be seen: (i) there is a slight tendency toward increased asymmetries, probably associated with unilateral control of midline organs in vocal communication; (ii) there is a strong tendency for increased communication between the left and right cerebral hemispheres – in fact, the increase in the number of commissural fibers is greater than the increase in cortical growth itself. Something is happening here in the 'horizontal' dimension which may give us some clues concerning the brain code!

In most people there is distinct and unequivocal asymmetry of function of the cerebral hemispheres with regard to speech and handedness. Given the importance of language in human life and the fact that linguistic manipulations preoccupy and demand from social beings so much time and energy, other functional asymmetries of the brain may very well be direct or indirect consequences of the language asymmetries. At the very least, we know that the left hemisphere is heavily involved in most of the major *expressive* functions – speech and the skilled use of the right hand. Whatever the exact nature of the right hemisphere's functions, the size and continuing growth of the corpus callosum suggests that right-hemisphere talents may be in some way complementary, rather than competitive or simply unrelated to left-hemisphere functions.

Most explanations of brain functions focus on the importance of the cerebral cortex – but is it accurate to speak of 'the cortex,' when we all in fact have *two cortices*? Historically the issue of the bilaterality of the nervous system and the conundrum of left and right and mirror-reversals have been little more than curious footnotes in the science of the brain – somehow too familiar to be of interest, too obvious to be profound. However, together with the relatively recent surge in interest in the talents of the right hemisphere, there has been a return to some of these fundamental questions concerning left and right. In the chapters which follow, we will see that the topic of 'the cortices' is both interesting and profound.

2

BRAIN STRUCTURES INVOLVED IN INTERHEMISPHERIC COMMUNICATION

The unusual functional asymmetry of the human brain poses several fascinating questions. Why are the human cerebral hemispheres so much more different from one another than the hemispheres of most other species? How does that asymmetry arise and how important is it for our characteristically human thought processes? Is evolution leading us toward complete asymmetry?

At least with regard to human speech and handedness, we can be certain that the left and right hemispheres in normal adults are *not* functionally identical. How can that be? Two possible answers are that either (i) the cerebral hemispheres are so markedly different in terms of their inherent structure that they 'think' differently, or (ii) there is an interhemispheric mechanism of communication which results in asymmetries of function.

Although these two possibilities are not mutually exclusive, they represent two distinctly different conceptions of brain organization. The idea that differences in the functioning of brain regions are due to large or small morphological differences is essentially a reductionist perspective, in which each portion of the brain (in this case, the left or right cerebral hemisphere) has unique functions attributable to *inherent neuronal wiring*. In this view, it is thought that each hemisphere will have certain kinds of internal connections or neuronal 'modules' which process information in ways not occurring contralaterally. In contrast, the idea that functional differences are due primarily to differences generated during the *interaction* of two brain regions can perhaps be characterized as a connectionist perspective. In this view, the process of information transfer itself – with or without inherent morphological differences between the regions – becomes an important factor in determining the functions of portions of the cortex.

To what degree the known anatomical asymmetries of the human brain can account for functional asymmetries will be discussed in chapter 3, but the approximate overall symmetry of the brain should be noted at the outset. Slight quantitative asymmetries can be found in brain specimens from several species (including the rat, cat, songbird and gorilla), but all brain structures except those located on the midline are found in pairs of roughly similar size. There are no *gross* structural asymmetries, such as seen in the heart or liver, and no *gross* developmental asymmetries which could establish an early functional asymmetry. A possible exception is the habenular nucleus – a small limbic system nucleus, which is divided into two subnuclei in the left hemisphere of man, but is a unitary structure on the right. Nevertheless the bilateral symmetry of the brain is so complete that, among the major internal organs, only the kidneys show as strong a tendency for bilaterally symmetrical organization as the brain!

The reality of some small anatomical asymmetries, discussed in chapter 3, may be an important factor in the emergence of a speech-dominant hemisphere, but it is not unreasonable to suspect that there might be a dynamic relationship between the cerebral hemispheres which also plays a role in the emergence of different modes of cognition. In other words, the transmission of nervous impulses across fibers connecting the two halves of the brain may be partly responsible for the differences in hemispheric function.

It is unlikely that theoretical arguments would allow us to choose unambiguously between the reductionist and connectionist perspectives, but it is worth noting the directions in which these two views lead. On the one hand, a hypothesis concerning inherent morphological asymmetries of the brain can be empirically tested in terms of the gross anatomy of cortical lobes, gyri, sulci, cerebral blood vessels or other macroscopic features of the brain. Alternatively asymmetries can be searched for in terms of fine-grained cellular asymmetries of a yet unknown kind or differences in neurotransmitter abundance. Regardless of which of several levels are to be scrutinized, the empirical search from the reductionist perspective focuses on crucial subcomponents which are presumed to bias the functioning of the system as a whole.

In contrast, from the connectionist perspective the empirical task is primarily to find mechanisms of communication which could result in functional differences. This research program can be pursued in terms of the dynamic relationships among neurons at a cellular level and in terms of relatively macroscopic electrical or metabolic activity, using the electroencephalograph (EEG) or more sophisticated techniques. Moreover, unlike the reductionist program, which relies entirely on investigations on organic tissue, the connectionist approach can make use of systems theoretical methods and computer simulations to identify possible relationships among known brain elements (see appendix 2).

As a rule, scientists prefer the reductionist methodology and most of science can be characterized as a process of searching for and isolating the smaller pieces within complex systems, and then testing for the effects of changes wrought in those pieces. Reductionism has of course proven its value many times in science, but the complexity of the brain is such that the systems theoretical approach may contribute significantly here. While the gross morphological and fine cellular findings of reductionist science will undoubtedly remain the bedrock of our understanding of brain function, mathematical modeling and systems theoretical arguments may well lead to an understanding of the high-level functions of the brain which are not directly apparent from anatomical and physiological findings.

Regardless of which perspective we may feel to be more promising, an understanding of the main themes of brain anatomy is prerequisite to any understanding of brain function. Let us begin therefore with a sagittal (midline) cut between the human cerebral hemispheres – revealing the nervous structures which allow the two halves to communicate (figure 2.1).

Such gross dissection already provides some insight into how the brain is organized: the two massive cerebral hemispheres are connected primarily by one major tract, the corpus callosum. The upper brainstem shows relatively more abundant lateral connections – across several commissures, including the posterior commissure, the habenular commissure, a portion of the anterior commissure and the so-called thalamic adhesion (which is present in 70 percent of human brains). But not until we descend to the lower brainstem is it apparent that

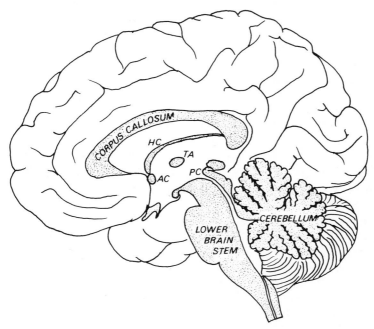

Figure 2.1 The medial aspect of the right hemisphere. A sagittal section between the cerebral hemispheres requires cutting all fibers which cross the midline (stipled regions). These include the corpus callosum and the anterior commissure (AC), which connect the left and right neocortices. The older parts of the cortex (paleocortex) and the diencephalon are joined by the hippocampal commissure (HC), the posterior commissure (PC) and the thalamic adhesion (TA). Various portions of the hypothalamus have bilateral connections, as does virtually all of the lower brainstem, including the cerebellum.

25

cross-talk is widespread and incessant, since virtually all portions of the lower brainstem, including the cerebellum, send and receive transverse fibers.

Given a somewhat unitary brainstem core, the brain can be conveniently subdivided into three principal structures: the midline brainstem, the neocortex of the cerebral hemispheres and the forebrain commissures – principally the corpus callosum – which connect the cortices (figure 2.2).

The neocortex

The neocortex of each hemisphere is a thin sheet of neurons approximately 1,600 cm^2 in area and 2–3 mm in thickness. It is called 'grey matter' because of the slightly darker appearance of nervous tissue which contains a high proportion of neuronal cell bodies. Beneath it lies the voluminous 'white matter,' consisting primarily of the connecting fibers which run short and long distances between cortical grey areas and to subcortical structures.

By recording from individual neurons of the cortex with a fine electrode, physiologists have discovered that cortical neurons lying in the same vertical dimension (perpendicular to the external surface of the brain) normally have similar electrical properties – responding to the same kinds of stimuli as their neighbors above and below. This is found to be the case throughout the thickness of the cortex. Close neighbors in the horizontal direction, however, will normally differ in their response if they are separated by more than 100 μm.

The significance of this 'columnar' structure will be discussed further on pp. 68–75, but it is important to note here that this type of organization leads conveniently to a two-dimensional view of cortical function. Although the brain as a whole is certainly a complex three-dimensional structure, in most contexts the cortical surface of the brain can be considered as a flat map without consideration of the details of cell layering in the vertical dimension. In other words, whatever localization of function and specialization of large or small sections of neocortex may exist, they exist over a two-dimensional cortical space and not layer by layer in the third dimension as well.

In reality the neocortex is a convoluted sheet twisted around on itself, the details of this three-dimensional structure being extremely important clinically. But we must make a distinction between the three-dimensional complexity – with its significant implications for the neurosurgeon – and the two-dimensional simplicity, which is conceptually the more valid view. Certainly if our primary aim is to come to an understanding of brain function, we would be wise to set aside all problems concerning the complex three-dimensional topology of the cortex and concentrate on the organization of the two-dimensional cortical map.

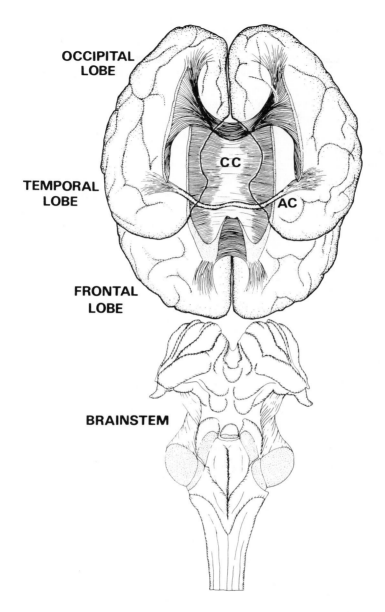

OCCIPITAL LOBE

TEMPORAL LOBE

CC

AC

FRONTAL LOBE

BRAINSTEM

Figure 2.2 The three principal structures of the brain: the midline brainstem, the cerebral hemispheres and the corpus callosum. The stipled areas on this posterior view of the brainstem indicate where the tracts leading to and from the cerebellum have been severed. The cerebral hemispheres have been up-ended to provide a view of the underside of the brain (after figure 149 of Nieuwenhuys *et al.*, 1978). The stipled regions on the corpus callosum (CC) indicate severance of callosal fibers that would otherwise extend to virtually all regions of neocortex. Note that the anterior commissure (AC) connects regions of anterior temporal cortex.

From this perspective, the diagrams of the brain found in most neurology textbooks are neither the easiest nor the most enlightening places to start. For example, as shown in figure 2.3, there may be much to learn from such illustrations concerning how the brain actually sits in the skull and what areas are likely to be affected by various forms of trauma, but they do little for our understanding of cortical organization. Where, for example, is the limbic system in figure 2.3? How is insular cortex related to the other cortical lobes? How can we conceptualize the fact that recently evolved 'neocortex' is six-layered, whereas the more ancient portions of cortex, the 'paleocortex,' is three-layered? Where is the hippocampus in all this?

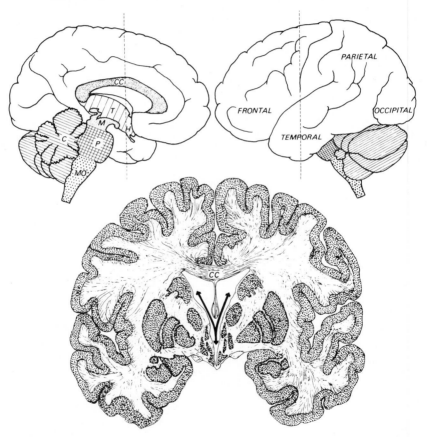

Figure 2.3 The gross anatomy of the brain. Shown above are medial and lateral views of the left hemisphere. Below is shown a cross-section of both hemispheres at the plane indicated by the dashed lines above. Key: CC, corpus callosum; T, thalamus; H, hypothalamus; M, midbrain; P, pons; C, cerebellum; MO, medulla oblongata. Note the position of the interventricular foramen (arrows) which is an opening connecting the lateral ventricles with the midline third ventricle. The third ventricle continues down the length of the spinal cord.

These questions would be far more easily answered if we could translate the convoluted three-dimensional structure into two dimensions. A two-dimensional map would not help the neurosurgeon in dissecting portions of the real brain, but such a map would be a useful starting-point in our attempt to understand where and how the brain stores and transmits information.

As illustrated in figure 2.4 translation into two dimensions can be accomplished by 'inflating' an elastic cerebral hemisphere like a balloon and then stretching the opening until the entire cortex is pulled into a two-dimensional plane. Our hypothetical elastic hemisphere can be inflated in this way through the so-called interventricular foramen, which is the opening through which the cerebrospinal fluid flows from the midline third ventricle into the lateral ventricles of each cerebral hemisphere. An inflated left hemisphere would then appear as seen in figure 2.4(A). If we now stretch the cingulate-limbic cortex out (as shown in figure 2.4(B)), we can produce a two-dimensional map of the entire cortex of one cerebral hemisphere.

As shown in figure 2.5, if the known relative positions and relative areal measures of the various sulci and gyri are maintained, it is then possible to get a clear idea of the planar structure of the cortex, without the topological confusions which the neurosurgeon is well paid to understand.

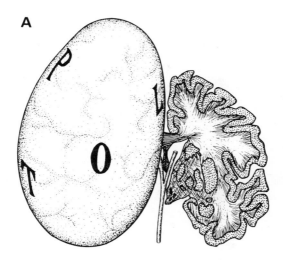

Figure 2.4 The construction of a two-dimensional brain map. A shows an inflated left hemisphere. By removing the white matter and all subcortical tracts and nuclei from the left hemisphere, and then 'inflating' it via the interventricular foramen, a smooth cortical surface is produced (B). Having inflated the left hemisphere, severed all commissural fibers, and removed all subcortical tissue, the cortical 'balloon' can be laid flat by stretching the opening of the interventricular foramen. The various cortical lobes are: P, parietal; O, occipital; T, temporal; I, insular; L, limbic.

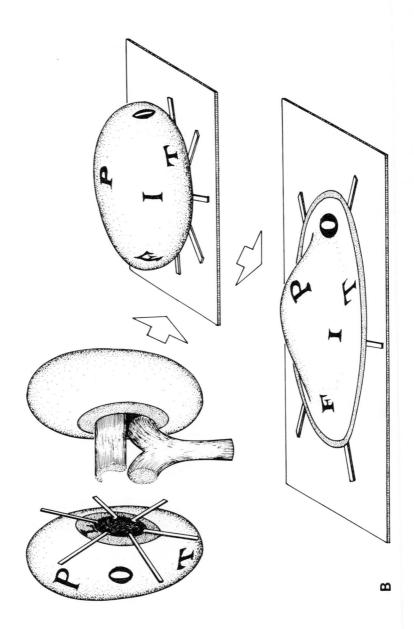

B

Of particular interest in this view of the cortex is the position of the so-called limbic lobe. Broca originally called this part of the brain 'limbic' because it formed a border or 'limbus' around the brainstem. Depicted as a flat cortical map, however, it can also be seen that the limbic lobe forms a border around the neocortex. In this view the three-layered limbic cortex is a midstation between the six-layered neocortex and the specialized ganglia of the brainstem, which receive their strongest cortical input from the 'heart' of the limbic system, consisting of the hippocampus, septum and amygdala. This is hardly a major discovery, but how many neurosurgeons, much less psychologists, appreciate the midway anatomical position of the limbic lobe!

The anatomical relationship between the insular cortex and the limbic lobe is also evident in figure 2.5. On both phylogenetic and cytoarchitectural grounds, the insula is more accurately described as

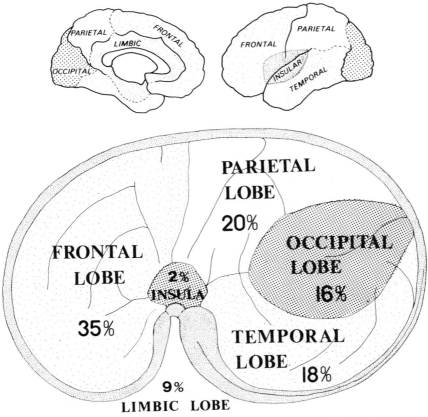

Figure 2.5 The two-dimensional cortical map and the more usual three-dimensional figure. The percentages of the total cortical surface area are also noted. (Further details are provided in appendix 1.) The six-layered neocortical top-hat has a three-layered limbic brim.

31

paleocortex, like most of the limbic lobe, than neocortex. In the two-dimensional cortical map, it is evident that the insula, together with the limbic lobe, forms a complete rim around the neocortex.

Needless to say there are various networks of corticocortical and cortico-subcortical fibers which allow for direct communication between distant brain regions, but insofar as there are 'mass-action' effects upon a region of cortex from its neighboring regions, this unusual map of the brain may tell us something not evident in the neurosurgeon's repair manual. In other words, if localization of function and spatial contiguity have any significance at all for cortical organization, then the two-dimensional cortical map may be the fundamental material from which a theory of brain function must be fashioned.

Given that the neocortex is best described as a flat map, our next question is to ask what kinds of sensory information are stored on it? Without getting side-tracked by too many of the interesting controversies in neurophysiology, let us first review some of the basic facts about the transmission of environmental stimuli to the brain.

How the brain sees: retinotopic maps
For over a century it has been known that localized regions of the cerebral cortex have limited functions. Although the degree of 'localizability,' or conversely the degree of 'equipotentiality' of the cortex, remains controversial, gross anatomy and early experimental techniques showed that there are some distinct differences in function among, notably, visual, somatosensory, auditory and motor cortex. The further demonstration of language-related areas by Broca and Wernicke strongly suggested that even 'higher' functions of the nervous system can be localized to subregions of the cortex, but the mechanisms of information storage and transfer remained completely unknown until the 1950s when microelectrode studies of nerve cells became possible.

Recordings from individual cells in the retina of the eye demonstrated that certain cells fire when struck by sufficient light. Moreover the activity of nearby cells is inhibited by their firing neighbors, suggesting the functional interconnection of neighboring cells. The outstanding feature of retinal physiology – which is now known in impressive detail – is that retinal stimulation with visible light produces biochemical changes (a conformational change in rhodopsin) which, in turn, increases the resting potential of retinal nerve cells, ultimately leading to action potential firing and the transmission of a nervous impulse from one nerve cell to others in the brain. Elucidation of the biochemistry and neurophysiology of this process must rank as one of the great achievements of twentieth-century science, but the central implication for psychology is simply but profoundly that photic stimuli can be transformed from the external world of electromagnetic physics into the internal world of neuronal chemistry.

The retina was soon understood to be a large mosaic of receptor cells with well-defined sensitivities and with, moreover, some relatively simple relationships among nearest neighbors: a center of activation would inevitably imply a surround of inhibition (figure 2.6(A)).

The information which is stored in patterns of activated and inactivated retinal cells was evident from macroscopic neuroanatomy to be transmitted to the brain along the optic nerve and tract to the lateral geniculate nucleus (LGN) of the thalamus. Again, single-cell studies have demonstrated the actual pattern in which this part of the brain stores the retinal image. Because the approximate relationships among various parts of the retina are maintained in the thalamus, the topographical pattern of visual stimulation is called 'retinotopic.' Of considerable interest here was the discovery that the individual retinal elements combine to have complex effects in the thalamus. That is, instead of a point-to-point correspondence between the retina and the thalamus, there is now a 'line-to-point' translation in which several excited cells lying on a line on the retina will together excite a 'simple' thalamic cell – the latter cell then storing information means a 'short line' or 'bar' of photic excitation (figure 2.6(B)).

It should be noted that the convergence of simple cell axons on complex cells (and complex cell axons on hypercomplex cells) can in fact occur within the retina itself in some species. Both for simplicity of exposition and because of the approximate validity in man, the first three stages of visual information processing will be discussed in terms of the retina, thalamus and striate cortex, but a completely unambiguous anatomical staging is not found.

This mechanism of information transfer illustrates two extremely important points about the brain. First, *there is a general topographical correspondence between a region of stimulation of the sensory organ and its representation in the central nervous system:* the location in the external visual field will translate directly to a region on the retina, and that retinal region will translate to a topographically related region of the thalamus. Secondly, *while maintaining topographical coherency, the nature of the information stored in the brain can change as it progresses from one way-station to the next.* The information at the thalamus (a bar of visual excitation) is stored not as the sum of its points (points of retinal excitation, ABC), but as an independent neural unit, a 'simple' cell, D. Although the pattern of thalamic neuronal activity is called 'retinotopic,' it is a more complex form of information storage than a centrally transplanted retina. It is, so to speak, the thalamus's 'interpretation' of the retinal image, with the basic geography of the retina maintained intact.

It is noteworthy that the translation from points ABC to bar D is unidirectional. Decoding D into its one-dimensional components would require additional neuronal machinery to trace the neuronal antecedents – machinery which is not inherent to the encoding process.

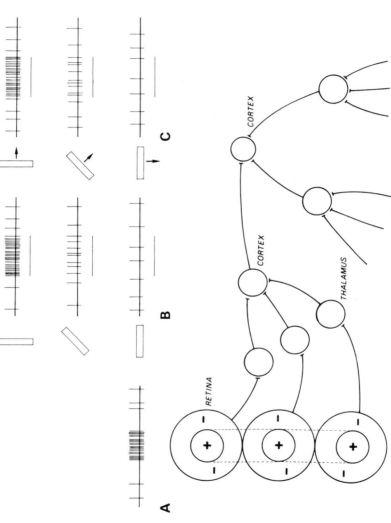

Fig. 2.6 The detection of points, lines and planes in the visual system. Part A shows the response of retinal cells to photic stimulation; B shows the response of a thalamic cell when several of its linearly aligned inputs are excited; C shows the response of a complex cell when several of its bar detector inputs are activated.

This fact is a simple manifestation of the unidirectionality of nervous impulses.

If retinal information storage can be characterized as a collection of points and that of the thalamus as a collection of bars, then it can be said that, on the visual cortex, information is stored as moving bars (= planes). Whereas the activity of a retinal cell would depend upon the amount of photic stimulation from a given point in the visual field, the activity of a neuron in the thalamus would depend upon the combined activity of several retinal cells along a short line in the visual field. At primary visual cortex, it is the movement of a bar of light in a particular direction which will be the factor deciding the amount of activity in a so-called 'complex' cell (figure 2.6(C)).

Starting with the patterns of cellular activity on the retina and tracing backward through the visual system, it has become known that visual information is stored as a spatial pattern of excited and inhibited neurons on the cerebral cortex and, moreover, that such information can be transmitted *in its entirety* to a second region by means of a set of essentially parallel nerve fibers. By recording the electrical responses of individual neurons from visual cortex subsequent to photic stimulation, it has become possible not only to map out the correspondence between retinal stimulation and cortical representation, but also to define the nature of the information being transmitted. Brightness, color, direction of stimulus movement and other characteristics of visual stimuli can be stored separately or in combination in cortical neurons.

As illustrated in figure 2.7 the 'retinotopic map' of the visual field is transmitted in this way from the retina to the lateral geniculate body (LGN) in the thalamus and from there to the primary visual cortex (striate cortex). Although there are gross distortions in these three visual maps, the relative positions of elements in the visual field are maintained at each level of neural organization. In other words, despite the radical change from light of various wavelengths and intensities to excitations of various classes of neuron and despite changes in the number of neural elements responsible for storing the visual information, the essential pattern remains unaltered as it is transmitted from the back of the eyeball to the back of the brain!

The actual storage of visual information in the brain is in fact more complex than might be assumed from the analogy with the lenses and mirrors of photographic equipment. The information stored at each location in visual cortex is dependent upon four factors concerning the impinging light stimulus – the location, intensity, color and orientation of the light in the visual field. Any given cell in visual cortex may store information concerned with one or several of these characteristics, so that the entire visual image must be built from a large number of cells containing such bits of information in order to avoid a disjointed, piecemeal view of the visual field. The complexity of the 'retinotopic map' is greatly increased as the information in the individual 'simple'

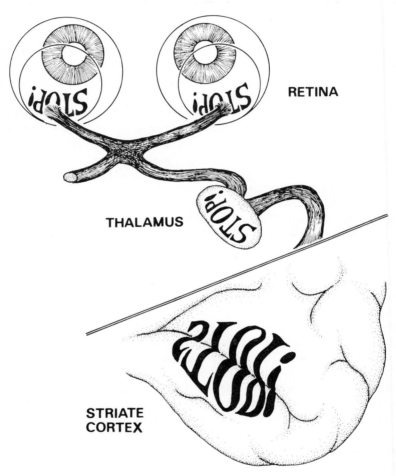

Figure 2.7 The primary 'retinotopic' map. In the visual system, the retinal image in the eye maintains its basic configuration as the pattern of stimulation is transferred from the retina to the lateral geniculate body in the thalamus to striate cortex. In the human brain, the central one or two degrees of the visual field (5–10 mm wide at a reading distance of 45 cm) is represented bilaterally.

cells are joined together in 'complex' and 'hypercomplex' cells. How the cortex manages to synthesize these individual quanta of information into a unified visual image, which appears to us as a complete and continuous representation of the external world, remains an unanswered question, but the map-like nature of the encoding in area 17 of primary visual cortex is well established.

Portions of the retinotopic map found in striate cortex are reproduced at least twice more in secondary visual cortex (areas 18 and 19). Unlike the mechanism of transfer from the retina to the cortex, however, the reproduction of the striate cortex pattern on to neighboring cortex results in a mirror-image reversal of the given pattern (figure 2.8). This inversion of the retinotopic map is an inevitable consequence of the anatomy of the so-called arcuate (arching or U-shaped) fibers which connect neighboring regions of cortex.

As is evident in figure 2.8, already it can be seen that the neat isomorphism between the pattern of stimuli at the body surface and the pattern stored in the brain has become complex. First, the visual image in the brain is split into two slightly overlapping halves in the two cerebral hemispheres and then it is divided into superior and inferior sections as the visual map is sent to secondary cortical regions.

As might be expected, the increasing topological complexity of the 'maps' of the visual field with increasing distance from primary sensory areas has led to discussion of the possibility of 'non-topographical' cortical representations (Phillips et al., 1984). In one sense this is obvious and inevitable. Insofar as color alone, texture alone, direction of movement alone or some partial representation of the retina is mapped on to secondary or tertiary sensory areas, 'retinotopic isomorphism' will soon suffer. Instead of a cortical representation of the 'flying sparrow,' there may be mapped only 'movement across the visual field' or 'decreasing intensity of central stimulus,' etc. It must be emphasized, however, that the 'topographical' nature of such high-level information will nonetheless be maintained – at least in the sense that the cortex is a two-dimensional sheet sending and receiving information to and from anatomically fixed regions. This is not to say that there will recur complete and precise retinotopic images all over the cortex. Rather, whatever form high-level information is stored in, it must be stored at cortical locations related to its informational content. Its spatial representation on the cortex will inevitably be one important aspect of cortical information storage.

Studies primarily on cats and monkeys have shown that some form of retinotopic organization is maintained in at least ten separate 'maps' in visual cortex (Merzenich and Kaas, 1980) – some of which are shown in figure 2.9. The labeling of such maps remains inconsistent among research groups and for different animal species, and it is simply unclear what portions of the occipital lobe should be called 'primary' and what portions 'secondary' or 'tertiary' visual areas. Regardless, it is worth

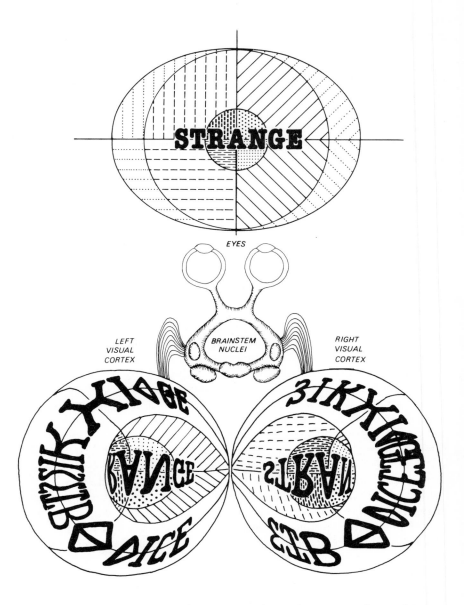

Figure 2.8 A schematization of the projection of a visual image on to the visual cortex of the left and right cerebral hemispheres. The retinotopic map in area 17 of each hemisphere is divided in two along the calcarine sulcus (corresponding to the horizontal equator of the visual field) and each half is separately projected to area 18 and again to area 19. The visual information is certainly 'topographical,' but no longer a straight-forward and complete representation of the visual field. The map is already upside down due to the effects of the corneal lens, and it is twice reversed left to right, resulting in the normal left-right (but upside-down) representation on the cortex.

emphasizing that an extremely large percentage of occipital cortex is involved in the construction of such maps.

THE BRAIN'S BODY IMAGE: SOMATOTOPIC MAPS

Since the cutaneous surface of the human body can itself be considered as a two-dimensional map, its representation on the two-dimensional cortex is most easily understood by first producing a map of the skin similar to that which the brain must deal with. This can be done by inflating the 'dermal bag' we all wear (figure 2.10) and then laying it flat with an incision along the spine (figure 2.11). Not shown in these maps is, of course, the internal surface of the gut which extends from within the mouth down to the anus, that is, the inner surface of the human 'tube' which is paradoxically also on the 'external' side of the body.

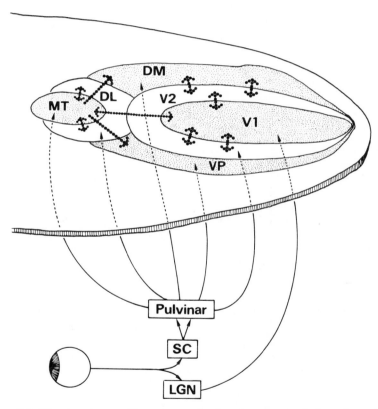

Figure 2.9 Visual pathways. The primary visual pathway proceeds from the retina, through the lateral geniculate nucleus (LGN) and goes to 'primary' visual cortex (V1), but other pathways traverse the superior colliculus (SC) and pulvinar (P) – giving rise to at least ten partial, but distinctly retinotopic maps on the monkey cortex. Note the abundance of reciprocal connections (↔) among the various maps. Key: DL, dorsolateral map; DM, dorsomedial map; MT, medial temporal map; V2, the 'secondary' visual map; VP, ventroposterior map.

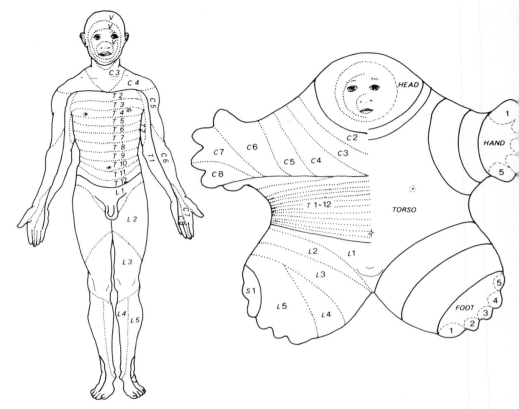

Figure 2.10 The inflated cutaneous 'bag.' To obtain an understanding of the nature of the sensory surface which the cortex must map, the human skin can be inflated to produce a nearly smooth surface. The regions covered by the various spinal nerves are: C, cervical; T, thoracic; L, lumbar; S, sacral. Sensory innervation of the face is primarily through the three branches of cranial nerve V (the trigeminal nerve).

Although we may be forgiven for not normally envisaging ourselves as skin balloons, the brain has the unhappy task of mapping this odd and lumpy cutaneous surface on to a two-dimensional cortical surface. As seen in figure 2.11, already our normal body sense – and possibly self-esteem – is radically altered in the two-dimensional map, but two further transformations occur as somatosensory information is sent to the brain.

First, there is considerable magnification of those skin regions which play an important role in tactile sensation of the external world. This distortion is due solely to the differences in density of nerve endings at various sites on the skin – an extremely high density of receptor organs on the fingers, toes, genitals and lips, and a relatively low density of receptors on the back of the head, trunk of the body and legs. There are, moreover, some slight twists and distortions – not unlike those found in the visual system – as the skin surface is mapped on to the cortex. Specifically, when representing one half of the map as shown in figure 2.11 (B) on the cortex, the genitals are found contiguous with the toes, rather than the torso, and the face is contiguous with the hands and fingers, rather than the back of the head and neck.

These distortions may strike us as bizarre, but given the ungainly surface of the human body to begin with, some such distortions are inevitable. For the skeptic who might think that the brain has done a poor job of mapping its body, just try to draw a sensible two-dimensional map of a doughnut – much less one with arms and legs!

If somewhat bizarre, the sequence of body regions shown in figure 2.11 does make sense as one possible solution of the cortical representation of the cutaneous map – particularly if there is some need to put the genitals and intra-abdominal regions near to limbic cortex (cingulate and insular cortex respectively). There is, however, one discontinuity in terms of the sequence of spinal nerves which remains unexplained. That is the sequence of spinal nerves entering the spinal cord at each of the vertebrae would be a natural sequence for subsequent cortical mapping, but strict adherence to this order is not found at the cortex. As shown in figure 2.11(B) the sequence of the *cervical* nerves has been reversed, relative to other spinal nerves, such that the first thoracic nerve (T1) is adjacent to the first cervical nerve (C2) rather than the last cervical nerve (C8). The significance of this reversal is unclear.

At any rate, the seemingly strange somatotopic map found on somatosensory cortex is strange primarily because of the inherent difficulty of producing a two-dimensional map of the body surface and not because of any perversity of the brain. It might also be mentioned in passing that the 'homunculus'-depiction of the body surface (the little man with large lips and huge hands appearing in most texts on the brain) is a misleading anthropomorphism. The three-dimensional 'homunculus' is a fiction, whereas the two-dimensional somatosensory map is a cortical reality.

The somatotopic maps are in fact cortical representations of various kinds of tactile sensation received over the entire surface of the body (and at least part of the internal gastrointestinal tract). As illustrated in figure 2.12, the somatotopic maps are transferred from the body surface via the thalamus (the ventral posterior nuclei) to a specific portion of the neocortex – the postcentral gyrus of the parietal lobe. In this region at least seven maps of the contralateral body surface (including representations of muscular sensation and joint sensation) are produced, each map representing slightly different aspects of tactile sensation (Merzenich and Kaas, 1980). In several primate species, and therefore probably in man as well, the most anterior somatosensory map (in area 3a) is concerned with perception of stimulation of the muscles. Immediately posterior in area 3b is the 'primary' map of cutaneous and muscle sensation. Behind that is area 1 with a map of cutaneous sensation

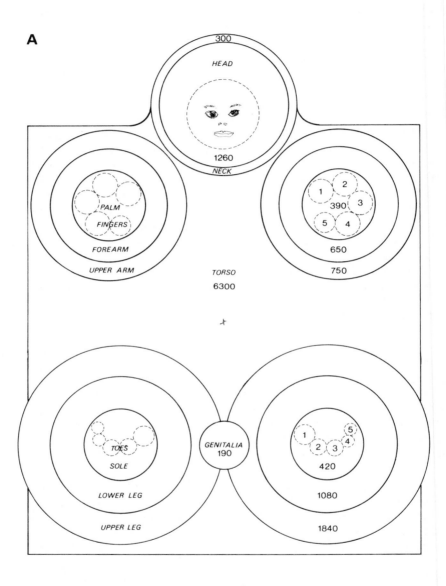

Figure 2.11 The two-dimensional cutaneous map. The numbers (other than those on the fingers and toes) denote the surface areas of the various regions (mm²). A typical 175 cm (5 foot 9 inch) man has approximately 18,300 mm² (2,840 sq. in) of surface

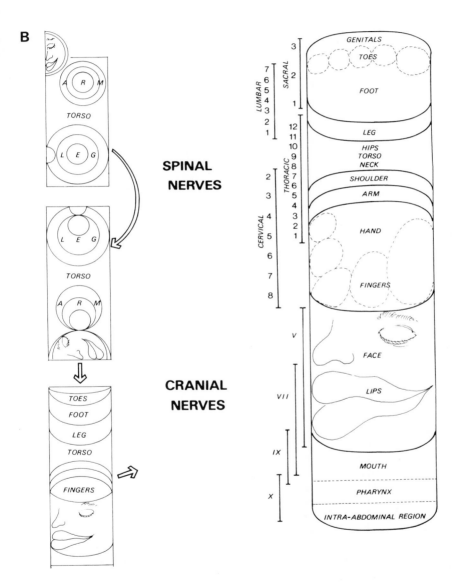

B

SPINAL NERVES

CRANIAL NERVES

area. Cutting the dermal map in half, turning it upside down and making some further distortions gives us the body map as found at somatosensory cortex (B). Note the reversed sequence of the cervical nerves.

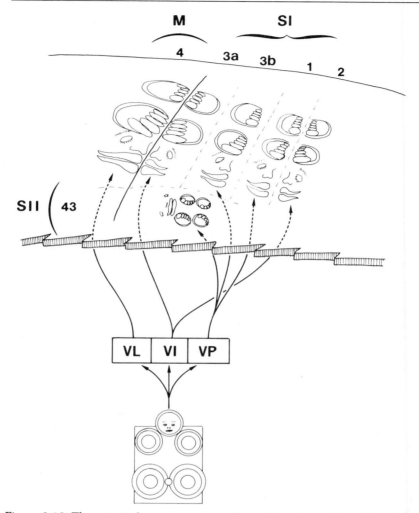

Figure 2.12 The principal somatosensory pathway. From the surface of the body, tactile information from skin, muscle and bone joints reaches the brain via the spinal and cranial nerves. The first way-station is in the thalamus (the ventrolateral nucleus (VL), ventroinferior nucleus (VI) and the ventroposterior nucleus (VP)), where somatotopy is maintained, and the second is the parietal neocortex (area SI). A second region of cortical somatotopy (area SII) is found closer to temporal cortex.

alone, followed by area 2 with skin and joint sensation. In area 5 behind area 1, there is a map of skin, muscle, periosteal and deep joint sensation. Finally, toward the insula, there is yet another somato-sensory pattern (SII) with apparently exaggerated representations of the mouth, tongue and perhaps visceral organs.

Taken as a whole, the pattern of somatosensory information storage in the parietal lobe appears to be even more complex than the patterns in visual cortex, since the various submodalities of 'touch' are arranged in narrow strips rather than as a single overlapping 'primary map,' such as found in area 17 of visual cortex. Similar to the visual map, however, there are at least two stages of increasing complexity which have led to convenient, if somewhat inaccurate, labels of 'primary' and 'secondary' somatosensory areas. It appears, therefore, that – just as the complexity of visual information increases as we move from area 17 through 19 – the complexity of somesthetic representations increases as we move posteriorly from area 3b toward 7.

Somatosensory information is stored in the cortex posterior of the central sulcus, but it is of interest that a similar and anatomically related topographical map of the musculature of the entire body is also found anterior of the central sulcus and again further anteriorly in premotor cortex. Unlike the somatosensory maps, the somatomotor maps are involved directly in the motor control of the striate musculature of the body.

It is therefore clear that, while difficult questions may remain concerning the nature of the information processing subsequent to somatosensory mapping and prior to somatomotor mapping, two-dimensional 'maps' are the starting and finishing points for somato-sensory perception and somatomotor action *at the cortical level*. The brain uses two-dimensional maps to perceive the world and to act on it.

How the brain hears: tonotopic maps

Auditory sounds are translated from changes in the density of molecules in the air into nervous impulses at the cochlear membranes (figure 2.13). As with touch and sight, the majority of auditory nerve fibers from each ear ascend to the contralateral cerebral hemisphere, although more ipsilateral 'leakage' is allowed in the auditory system.

The mapping of auditory frequencies undergoes several trans-formations in the auditory pathway. A sound of given frequency is represented by a single point in the cochlea, by a two-dimensional sheet of cells in the auditory nuclei and by a one-dimensional strip of cells on the primary cortex. Orthogonal to the isofrequency bands are 'binaural response-specific bands' (Middlebrooks et al., 1980). What this means is that while the tone (frequency) of a sound will determine the location of its cortical representation in one dimension, the second dimension of the tonotopic map will be concerned with the relative input from the ears (the location of the sound relative to the midline of the body) (see figure 2.14).

Again it is primarily the mechanisms of the pre-cortical processing which excite the physiologist – and which have the most significance for clinical medicine – but it is the two-dimensional cortical represen-tation which is of interest to the psychologist. Having traversed four brainstem nuclei (the cochlear nuclei, the olivary nuclei, inferior colliculus and the medial geniculate body), auditory information

45

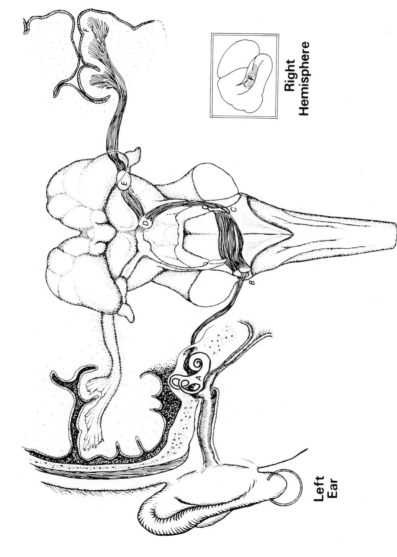

Right Hemisphere

Left Ear

Figure 2.13 The auditory system. Sound waves are translated into nervous impulses at the cochlea (A) and brought to auditory cortex (F) over four processing stations: B, the cochlear nuclei; C, the olivary nuclei; D, the inferior colliculus; E, the medial geniculate body.

reaches the cortex and again is mapped in two dimensions. At least six such maps have been identified in the auditory cortex of the monkey, and the precision of the mapping appears to be as great or greater than that found in visual cortex (Merzenich and Kaas, 1980).

Because the information stored in temporal cortex is auditory in nature and not visual, it is less easily visualized than that stored in visual cortex, but the organizational principles are similar. The basic configuration of the mapping in the primary auditory field is by the sound frequency in one dimension and by alternating strips of bilateral and unilateral cochlear representation in the other dimension. In primary auditory cortex (AI), higher frequencies are mapped anteriorly and lower frequencies posteriorly (although this pattern is reversed in secondary auditory fields). In the dimension orthogonal to frequency, the alternating layers of bilateral and unilateral representation allow for identification of the source of the sound. That is, whereas strong input to one ear and weak input to the other ear will indicate a source far to one side of the head, approximately equivalent inputs to both ears will indicate a midline source.

Again we find that – at the first cortical stage – the cortex stores information concerning a time-varying three-dimensional world as a two-dimensional map (figure 2.14). Undoubtedly because of the importance of the temporal dimension in hearing, the cortical map of the auditory field strikes us as particularly abstract. Unlike a single frame of a visual 'movie' or an instantaneous map of the entire field of touch, a few milliseconds of sound provides us with very little high-level information. Several of the auditory maps must be brought together in sequence before we can determine, for example, the meaning of a spoken word or the speed of an approaching train. The fact that auditory 'meaning' therefore seems several steps away from the primary sensation may explain why the extent of 'primary' auditory cortex containing identifiable maps is so much smaller than those of touch and vision, despite the obvious importance of hearing for many animals, particularly man. Nevertheless, again we find that the first cortical representation of the auditory world is also a rather sensible two-dimensional map.

TWO-DIMENSIONAL MAPPING
Whereas light of various wavelengths and intensities is transformed in the visual system into the firing of cells which have positions in visual cortex related to the position of the light in the visual field, sounds of various frequencies and amplitudes are transformed in the auditory system into the firing of cells which have positions in auditory cortex related to the frequency and source of the sound in the auditory field.

In the case of somatosensory cortex it is easily understood that the information concerning the sensation on the two-dimensional skin surface would be translated into a two-dimensional cortical map. Even

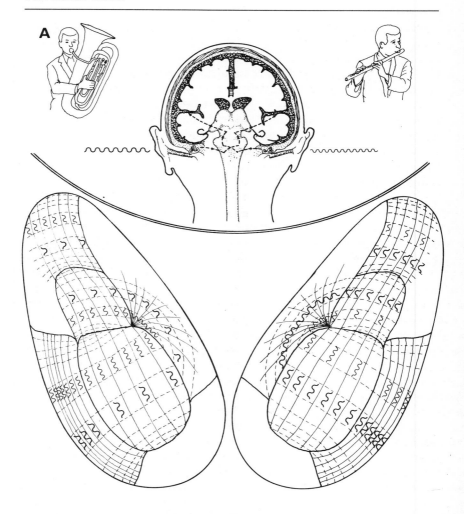

AUDITORY CORTEX

Figure 2.14 The tonotopic maps found on auditory cortex. (A) The auditory field is represented on the cortex in two orthogonal dimensions – one extending along the

in the case of 'deep' body sensations, where a two-dimensional description seems less accurate a representation of the sensory field, again a two-dimensional 'map' is the cortex's way of storing somatosensory information. For the visual modality a two-dimensional representation of the visual field is once again intuitively appealing, since the visual field can be thought of as a flat picture of the external world. For the auditory modality it is less obvious that a two-dimensional map would serve a useful purpose – not because hearing is more three-dimensional than sight or touch, but because the temporal dimension is so important

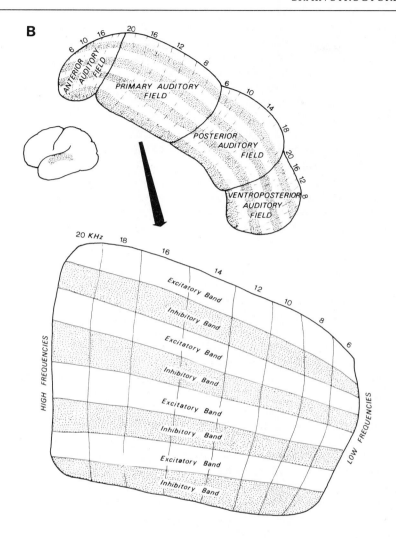

anterior–posterior axis, along which the frequency of sounds are mapped and one which maps the source of the sound in the auditory field relative to the midline. (B) Further details of the auditory maps.

for obtaining meaning from auditory signals. Nonetheless cortical maps on which sound stimuli are identified in terms of their x- and y-coordinates over appropriate cortical space is the way in which the cortex initially records auditory phenomena. Wavelengths and intensities of light, submodalities and intensities of touch and frequencies and amplitudes of sound are all transformed into the activity of neurons in a two-dimensional cortical world.

The mechanism of cortical information storage in auditory cortex is particularly instructive in one additional way. Since one of the major features of auditory information is the frequency of the sound stimulus, it might naively be thought that all the brain needs to do to record information concerned with sound frequencies is to have a cell which will fire at the same frequency as the external stimulus. Except in the case of extremely high frequency sounds, neurons are generally capable of firing rapidly enough to do so, but the cortex has clearly opted for a digital rather than an analog representation. Despite the fact that sounds can be described in terms of frequencies and amplitudes, cortical cells whose firing 'means' middle C do not themselves fire at rates related to the 261.63 vibrations per second which middle C is acoustically. On the contrary, cells whose firing corresponds to middle C can fire at any frequency without altering the acoustic meaning of that activity. The firing of middle C cortical neurons will always signify middle C − never G sharp or B flat because of changes in firing frequency. Only the perceived *intensity* of middle C will be affected by changes in the rate of cell firing.

But let us not get too wrapped up in questions of the neuron code!

The significance of these topographical maps for sight, sound and touch lies in the fact that − however it is that neurons are clever enough to transmit information from the body surface for storage in the brain − the brain ends up, first of all, with quite a few sensory 'maps' of the external world. At the latest count, twenty-three maps of the auditory, visual and somatosensory modalities have been identified in the monkey; if we include primary and secondary somatomotor maps and possible gustatory and olfactory maps, clearly a significant portion of the cortex is engaged in cartography of one kind or another.

Although there is a translation of sensory information from the physical units of the 'real world' into the jargon of neurons, in effect, we can say that there is an *excitatory* relay of external patterns of physical stimuli to related internal patterns at the cortex. For all kinds of sensory perception, inhibitory effects among nearest neighbors at each stage of processing are essential for allowing the transmission of well-defined stimuli to the brain, but the nature of the net effect should not be overlooked: an (auditory, visual or somesthetic) image of the external world is translated into a related topographical representation in the brain. Such *excitatory* mapping is unquestionably a major part of the brain code.

Given the reality of these diverse sensory (and motor) maps, the next question in approaching the brain code may simply be: How important are such maps? Certainly we can say that the cortex receives information about the external world in terms of such maps and appears to control somatic motor activity by making use of such maps, but what happens in between?

The traditional view has been that primary sensory and primary motor cortical representations encompass only a small percentage of the total cortical surface area, and that the percentage of cortex taken up by such maps decreases with phylogeny. As Merzenich and Kaas (1980) have recently pointed out, however, modern studies on the primate brain show that sensory 'mapping' is predominant over most of the posterior half of the primate brain. Areas that were once labeled as 'secondary' or 'tertiary' sensory cortical regions are now known to have sensory maps which are not merely representations of the primary sensory maps, but which themselves receive sensory input directly from the brainstem and have distinct topographical structure similar to the structure of 'primary' areas. Whether or not we should label such areas 'secondary sensory' or 'associational' is debatable, but it is important to recognize that, as real as higher-level abstract encoding may be, a significant portion of the brain is involved (simply!) in the representation of various aspects of the sensory field.

Debate continues whether or not sensory cortex is organized serially in regions with successively 'higher' functions, or in parallel with different functions at several regions of sensory cortex, but the trend of current research seems to favor the importance of the parallel processing view. Serial and parallel processing are not of course mutually exclusive. Although the vast amount of parallelism (the large number of sensory maps) has come as something of a surprise, there are undoubtedly serial effects as well. (See chapter 6 for some convincing anatomical evidence for the reality of serial processing.)

The traditional serial view has been that a very small primary sensory region is surrounded by secondary, tertiary and ultimately associative cortical regions, but particularly in visual cortex it is apparent that retinotopic maps are located over virtually all of the occipital lobe and extend into the temporal lobe. Somatotopic maps are now known to cover parietal lobe areas 3, 1, 2 and 5, and possibly part of 7 and insular cortex. Tonotopic maps occupy a more modest proportion of the temporal lobe, but the further identification of meaningful auditory dimensions may well lead to the discovery of other kinds of auditory maps in temporal cortex. The remaining posterior cortical regions may be fairly labeled 'association' cortex (areas 39 and 40 and much of the anterior temporal lobe), but these regions without known topographical maps constitute no more than 30 percent of the neocortex posterior of the central sulcus. For methodological reasons the rules for mapping in frontal cortex are less well known, but the topography of primary and supplementary motor maps is well understood.

It is worth noting, however, that the topographical configuration of remaining sensory cortical regions may well go undetected – not because of a lack of topography, but because of the small percentage of the sensory field which is mapped there. Certainly for human beings most visual information does not come from the periphery of the 180° visual field, but from our perceptions within the central 2–4° of the midline. We of course maintain a wide enough visual field of attention that we will notice the swerving bus or advancing lion in the peripheral field, but normally our evaluations of the wider world will be acted upon only once the peripheral stimulation has been brought within the central field (2–4°) for analysis. Similarly for touch, in which we rely heavily on the fingertips and lips for scrutiny of environmental objects. Although in an experimental situation we may be able to discriminate shapes and textures at many regions of the skin, we would never deliberately attempt to discriminate wool from cotton or an oily substance from a watery substance using our elbows!

Although more complex, our powers of auditory discrimination are also normally exercised over a much smaller range than our capabilities would allow. Not only are we more competent at discriminating middle-range frequencies, but also we characteristically position our heads to maximize the sound coming to both ears. We 'look at' any noise which we want to analyze. In other words, the auditory map of central importance is one which includes only the sound frequencies of normal speech with, moreover, approximately equivalent input from the two ears.

So although rather large sensory fields are mapped on to primary sensory cortex, much of our higher cognitive, discriminative and analytic powers are based upon information which is found in a very small subset of each modality map. What this may mean is that sensory or associative cortex which does not appear to contain a topographical map may simply contain a very large map of a very small spectrum of sensation, thus obscuring its inherent topography. Particularly when superimposed on a map from a second modality in the process of polymodal association, existing topographical maps may not be easily detected. At present what is known is that approximately 40 percent of the cerebral cortex stores topographical maps related to the perception of the internal and external worlds or motor activity within them.

The brainstem

The retinotopic, somatotopic and tonotopic maps at various regions of sensory cortex are the first indication how the brain can store and transmit information. Yet even if we were to assume that the cortex is involved solely in the construction and manipulation of such maps, much of the brain lies below the two-dimensional cortical umbrella and is anatomically not configured in such a way that many other such 'maps' are possible.

Indeed the brainstem is a thick 'stem' located on the midline of the brain beneath the white and grey matter of the cerebral hemispheres (see figure 1.1). It is usually characterized as being primarily (i) a bundle of sensory tracts – relaying (topographical) messages from the body surface to the cortex (the map-making routes); (ii) a bundle of motor tracts – relaying (topographical) messages from the cortex to the

somatic structure; (iii) a collection of nuclei which control the autonomic nervous system; and (iv) a network of tracts and nuclei which are
involved in attention and arousal.

Functions (i) and (ii) are fundamentally topographical – whether the
topographical maps contained within the thalamic nuclei or the
topography implicit to the tracts which connect peripheral receptors
with the thalamus. Such relay mechanisms are of only limited interest,
however, insofar as they represent nothing more than the precursors of
the cortical maps without additional information processing. Function
(iii) involves nuclei of the hypothalamus and lower brainstem. Their
functioning is essential for maintaining the physiological homeostasis of
the body, but insofar as these autonomic and neurosecretory nuclei are
essentially *effector* mechanisms, they are of limited relevance to the
brain code.[1] It is the fourth *nontopographic* property of the brainstem –
attention and arousal (iv) – which is of interest in the present context.

Although it is generally true that damage to any brain structure will
have multiple effects which are rarely confined to sensory, motor or
cognitive functions alone, nonetheless parcelation of the brainstem
into the predominant roles of its various subcomponents is again
heuristically useful. As shown in figure 2.15, the bulk of the lower part
of the brainstem is involved in sensory or motor functions. Starting
from the bottom and working up, the spinal cord consists predominantly of motor tracts running in the anterior half and sensory tracts running
in the posterior half of the cord. Above it the medulla oblongata is a
continuation of those tracts with a few crucial ganglia engaged in the
regulation of autonomic processes (breathing, heart-rate, etc.). Above
the medulla are the pons and metencephalon, containing progressively
more and more regions whose functions are neither solely motor nor
solely sensory. Above the mesencephalon lies the diencephalon,
containing two interesting structures, the hypothalamus (the 'head
ganglion' of the autonomic nervous system) and the thalamus (the first
major processing station for most sensory input).

What should be evident from figure 2.15 is the fact that the lower
brainstem at each of the depicted cross-sections is mostly involved in
the sending and receiving of information between the thalamus and the
peripheral sensor and effector mechanisms – functions (ii) and (iii).
Unlike the upper brainstem, only a relatively small part of the lower
brainstem is involved in functions (iii) and (iv).

At the level of the thalamus (figure 2.16) the so-called 'specific'

[1] The brain code, however, is of tremendous relevance to the functioning of the brainstem
and particularly the mechanisms of control over the autonomic nervous system. It is likely that the
patterns of input from neocortex and limbic cortex have significant influence on the activity of the
hypothalamus, in particular. Insofar as the hypothalamus is itself the central control station for
controlling the balance of the electrolytes of body fluids, regulating body temperature, heart-rate
and pituitary hormones, the question of where it receives its instructions is of obvious importance.
The translation rules from cortical maps to hypothalamic activity may someday constitute a central
dogma for the mechanisms of psychosomatic disorders.

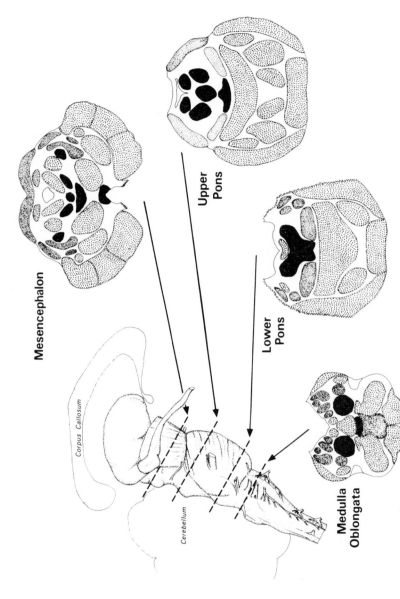

Figure 2.15 Sections through the brainstem reveal the major ascending and descending tracts traversing through it. The stipled regions are sensory and motor tracts and nuclei; the darkened regions are tracts and nuclei involved in the tonic and phasic aspects of cortical arousal.

Mesencephalon

Upper Pons

Lower Pons

Medulla Oblongata

Corpus Callosum

Cerebellum

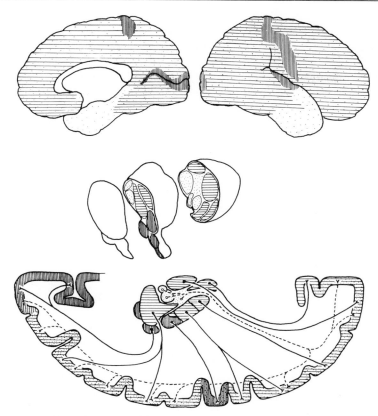

Figure 2.16 Gross dissection of the thalamus into three major subsystems – the sensory relay nuclei (vertically striped regions), the 'associational' nuclei (horizontally striped regions), and the nonspecific 'arousal' nuclei (stipled regions). Above and below are shown the cortical areas receiving thalamic output.

nuclei are predominantly sensory in nature and damage to them can lead to quite specific sensory deficits – auditory if the medial geniculate body is damaged, visual if the lateral geniculate body is damaged and somesthetic if the ventral posterior nuclei are involved. Yet those nuclei constitute only one relatively small part of the complex network of fibers connecting the brainstem to the cortex. The so-called 'non-specific' or 'association' nuclei of the thalamus send and receive far more fibers to and from the cortex – some 90 percent of the corticofugal and corticopetal pathways.

Notable is the fact that reciprocal connections between the thalamus and the cortex are extensive, but – in terms of the amount of thalamic tissue involved – the relaying of primary sensory data directly from the sense organs is a relatively minor function. Most of the thalamus is involved in activity which is best described as 'associational' – receiving

Table 2.1 The thalamic nuclei

Nucleus	Function	Cortical projections
Anterior nuclei	Association	Areas 23, 24
Medial nuclei	Arousal and attention	Areas 10, 11, 12, 47
Anterior ventral nuclei	Association	Areas 8, 9, 32, 44, 45, 46
Lateral ventral nuclei	Association	Areas 4, 6
Posterior ventral nuclei	Relay	Areas 1, 2, 3
Posterior ventral nucleus (pars parvocellular)	Relay	Area 43, Insula
Dorsal lateral nucleus	Association	?
Centromedian nucleus	Arousal and attention	? (primarily to other thalamic nuclei)
Parafascicular nucleus	Arousal and attention	? (primarily to other thalamic nuclei)
Lateral posterior nucleus and pulvinar	Association	Areas 5, 7, 39, 40, 18, 19, 37, 21, 22
Lateral geniculate nucleus	Relay	Area 17
Medial geniculate nucleus	Relay	Areas 41, 42

diverse inputs (often containing sensory information, but arriving via cortical or subcortical way-stations) and communicating with 'association' cortex. The diversity and complexity of these connections is made explicit in table 2.1.

As evident from both figure 2.17 and table 2.1, a large portion of the upper brainstem is not primarily sensory nor primarily motor, but rather is involved in yet poorly understood mechanisms of arousal, attention and association. So, setting aside all motor and sensory pathways, let us dissect the brain once more to see what structures below the cortex are involved in neither sensory nor motor, but 'associational', activities. By removing all tracts and ganglia which are defined classically as motor or sensory, we are left with the 'thinking' part of the brain – the cortex, corticocortical association fibers (including the corpus callosum) and all of the subcortical arousal and associational mechanisms (including a large part of the thalamus) (figure 2.17).

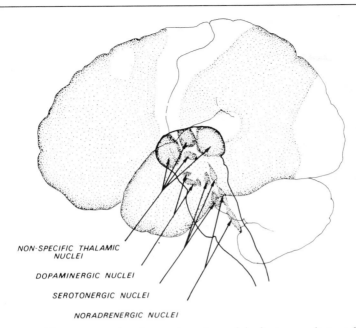

NON-SPECIFIC THALAMIC
NUCLEI

DOPAMINERGIC NUCLEI

SEROTONERGIC NUCLEI

NORADRENERGIC NUCLEI

Figure 2.17 The attentional and arousal portions of the brain – as distinct from the primary sensory and motor pathways.

The subcortical structures illustrated in figure 2.17 are of particular interest insofar as they constitute the neural mechanisms through which portions of cerebral cortex are aroused and conscious attention is brought to bear on information stored at a cortical level. The precise mechanisms and circuits involved are complex, but there is strong experimental evidence indicating that sensory information can be conveyed to the cortex via the normal primary sensory pathways – producing characteristic physiological responses (evoked potentials) at each stage along the way – but that sensory information will not reach conscious awareness *unless* there is sufficient neural activity within these subcortical arousal centers. Many anesthetic drugs which work on the central nervous system are thought to have their effects in this way: putting to 'sleep' the arousal centers and consequently blocking all sensory input from reaching consciousness, but not blocking the normal flow of sensory information along the primary sensory pathways.

Or more interest than the relatively long-term effects of brainstem 'arousal' mechanisms involved in sleep and anesthesia are the short-term effects involved in 'attention' and shifting attention. In the views of Crick (1984) and Robinson (1983), the role of the 'nonspecific' thalamic nuclei, and specifically the so-called 'reticular complex,' is to act as a 'searchlight' – selectively activating portions of the cortex. As recently reviewed by Crick (1984), this might be accomplished by means of the activation of relatively small portions of the corticothalamic/thalamocortical network, together with the simultaneous inhibition of other regions. This is likely to occur as follows: 'an active patch in the [reticular] complex [of the thalamus] will tend to suppress many other parts of the complex. . . . The effect will be to heat up the [more active,] warmer parts of the thalamus and cool down the [less active,] cooler parts.' This will produce positive feedback, such that 'attention' will be focused on the most highly activated thalamocortical region (Crick, 1984).

While detailed mechanisms remain uncertain, the brainstem has for decades been considered as the 'flywheel' of the central nervous system – capable of activating restricted parts of the brain. As such the communication from arousal centers to the cerebral cortex does not involve the flow of 'information,' in the sense that the topographical sensory maps contain 'information.' Arousal from sleep or a shift in attention from one topic to another can be thought of as simply activating cortical information which is already present.

In chapter 3 we will find that the central location of the brainstem is of importance for its functions as a 'flywheel.' Although it has approximate bilateral symmetry with connections primarily to its ipsilateral cerebral cortex, its massive network of internal cross-connections (particularly those of the so-called reticular activating system) means that its *dual searchlights* light up bilateral regions of cerebral cortex.

The corpus callosum

The third major component of the brain is the corpus callosum. It must be said that few books on the brain would elevate this commissure to such an exalted status (and many of the following pages are devoted to justifying this claim), but the anatomical justification is straightforward. While the cerebral cortex is involved (in the first instance) in the storage of sensory maps and the brainstem is involved in their selective activation and deactivation, corticocortical tracts (among which the corpus callosum is the largest) are involved in the process of association among the cortical maps. There are in fact some unusual features of the corpus callosum, but this tract is first and foremost a collection of corticocortical association fibers – and as such it is the largest tract devoted to intracortical communications.

It is difficult to estimate how much of the substance of the brain is involved in processes of corticocortical communications but, as depicted in figure 2.18, clearly we are not discussing some obscure nucleus in some faraway corner of the brain. At the very least, some 50 percent of the white matter of each cerebral cortex is allowing the cortex to talk with itself. The complexity of these fibers and the virtual impossibility of isolating them individually makes certain kinds of speculation about *intra*hemispheric association pointless, but here the corpus callosum is special. Traversing the gap between the cerebral hemispheres, the corpus callosum is exposed and provides a window on *inter*hemispheric cortical communication. It does not seem an unreasonable starting-point, therefore, to open the debate on intracortical communication with discussion of the corpus callosum.

Important for any theory of interhemispheric communications are the quantitative figures concerning both the cerebral cortex and the corpus callosum. The number of callosal fibers relative to the number of functional units of the cerebral cortex is particularly important, for these figures will give us some indication about the capacity of the corpus callosum to transmit cortical information from one side of the brain to the other. Let us therefore consider what is known about the areal extent of the cerebral cortex, the dimensions of the cortical columnar units which comprise it and current estimates concerning callosal size and termination.

The role of the anterior commissure will be discussed in chapter 6. Although it also is a forebrain commissure and is known to make roughly homotopic neocortical connections, in man it is approximately one-fiftieth the size of the corpus callosum and can therefore be discussed as a relatively minor aspect of interhemispheric relations.

As illustrated in figure 2.19 callosal fibers are known to connect most cortical regions. Portions of visual cortex (areas 17 and 18) have few callosal connections except those regions representing the vertical midline, and there is a paucity of callosal fibers connecting the hand and foot regions in somatosensory cortex, but all association cortical regions send and receive callosal fibers. The one exception is the association cortex near the temporal pole, but this region is bilaterally connected via the other major forebrain commissure, the anterior commissure.

The most important issue concerning the nature of the communications made possible by these commissures turns out to be that concerning which there is the greatest uncertainty, that is the number of callosal fibers. Estimates range from a figure of 1 million (Bailey and von Bonin, 1951, p. 240) through 250 million (Blinkov and Glezer, 1968) and beyond. This gross discrepancy can be partly resolved, however, if

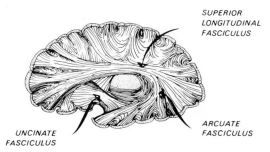

SUPERIOR
LONGITUDINAL
FASCICULUS

UNCINATE
FASCICULUS

ARCUATE
FASCICULUS

Figure 2.18 Three of the major intrahemispheric association pathways. Numerous other tracts allow for the distribution of cortical information to near and distant cortical sites.

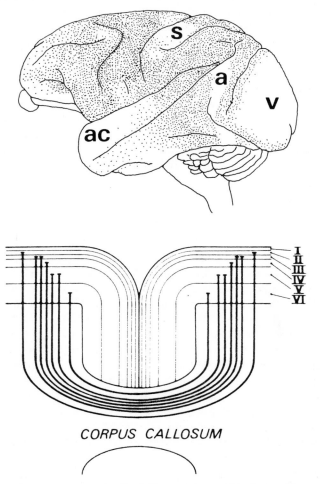

Figure 2.19 The termination of callosal fibers in the monkey brain. Above: Most of the cortex sends and receives callosal fibers. Regions that do not are the primary somatosensory (s), primary auditory (a) and primary visual (v) cortical areas. The temporal pole has commissural connections across the anterior commissure (ac) (modified from Myers, 1965). Below: In primates, callosal fibers start and finish at the same layer of neocortex (modified from Gazzaniga and LeDoux, 1978).

it is considered that Bailey and von Bonin's estimate of the diameter of individual callosal fibers (10 μm) was ten to twenty times that which has been reported subsequently (0.5–1.0 μm) (e.g. Fleischhauer and Wartenburg, 1967). If this latter figure concerning callosal fiber size is correct, then the Bailey and von Bonin figure must be increased by a factor of 100–400, i.e. to 100–400 million callosal fibers. Tomasch (1954) has also made an estimate in this range (200 million), but the largest figure comes from Myers (1965) who estimated that there are

700,000 fibers per square millimeter in the corpus callosum of the cat – a figure which would imply 490 million fibers in the human corpus callosum (7 cm^2 cross-section). As unsatisfactory as such diversity is, most researchers today accept that the number of callosal fibers is in the vicinity of 200–250 million (Garey, 1979; Doty and Negrao, 1973).

With regard to the number of structural and functional subunits of the cerebral cortex, there is at least some consensus that both structurally and functionally there are columnar units containing 1,000 to 100,000 neurons. Von Economo (1929) noted that such functional subunits are apparent in the cortex, and Lorente de No (1938) stated explicitly that the cortex may be organized into cylindrical columns which constitute both structural and functional units.

> All the elements of the cortex are represented in [cortical barrels] and therefore it may be called an elementary unit, in which, theoretically, the whole process of transmission of impulses from the afferent fiber to the efferent axon may be accomplished.

Lorente de No found these cylindrical units to be between 100 and 500 μm in diameter.

Since 1957 Mountcastle has been advocating a similar 'modular unit' conception of the cortex. The concept of the 'cortical column' which he and Hubel and Wiesel have popularized is, however, somewhat ambiguous in so far as the term 'column' has been used to mean: (i) a fundamental structural unit (or 'minicolumn' – Mountcastle, 1978); (ii) a somewhat larger structural unit of varying size depending upon the area of cortex (or 'macrocolumn' – Mountcastle, 1978); and (iii) a functional unit which is not necessarily identical to either the mini-column or the macrocolumn (Szentagothai, 1978a).

Generally speaking the minicolumn has been considered as the minimal anatomical unit of the cortex, whereas the macrocolumn has been considered to be a physiological unit of larger dimensions and which is perhaps divisible, depending upon the function under consideration. Let us consider both columnar units in turn.

Based upon the anatomical studies of Rockel *et al.* (1980), Mountcastle has argued that the minicolumn is a cylinder of neurons with a constant diameter of 30 μm. With the exception of striate cortex, where the cell number rises to approximately 260, the cell number within such minicolumns shows considerable constancy at around 110. This was found by Rockel *et al.* to hold true regardless of which neocortical area was examined (motor, somatosensory, frontal, parietal or temporal) and regardless of mammalian species (mouse, cat, rat, rhesus monkey or man). Since there are known differences in the thickness of the cortex according to species and area, the consistency of cell number across most areas indicates that there are differences in cell packing density, but not differences in the fundamental cellular components (see figure 2.20).

61

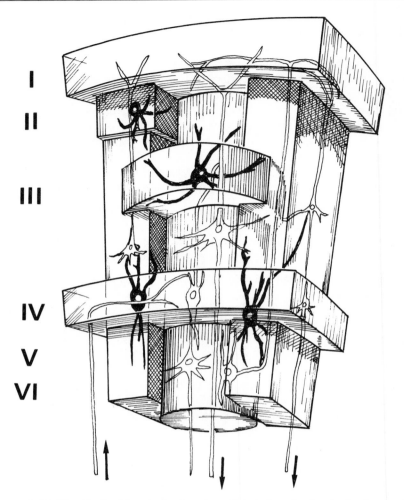

I

II

III

IV

V

VI

Figure 2.20 The idealized 'cortical column' – widely believed to be the fundamental computational unit of the cortex. Most incoming and outgoing fibers are excitatory (unshaded neurons), but many of columnar neurons (shaded) have inhibitory effects within the column and on nearest neighbors.

In striate cortex the dimensions of the minicolumns are the same as those of the ocular dominance columns and they are thought likely to be the same units (Mountcastle, 1978). Elsewhere in the brain, functional units vary from 50–60 μm in diameter (auditory cortex) to 200–300 μm (somatosensory cortex) to 500–1,000 μm (motor cortex). Moreover, columnar organization of the termination of callosal fibers has also been found, where again the diameters of the columnar units is between 200 and 500 μm (Goldman and Nauta, 1977). Characteristics of these columnar units are summarized in figure 2.21.

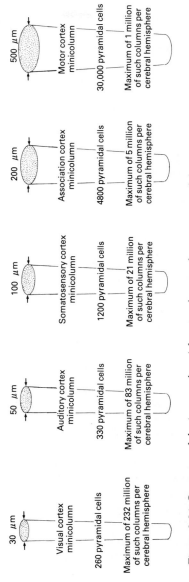

Figure 2.21 Summary of the 'macrocolumn' functional units of various parts of the cortex.

Based upon these anatomical considerations together with estimates of overall cortical area, rough estimates of the number of cortical columns in the human cortex are easily made. It should be said at the outset that such estimates are necessarily approximate, but they do give some idea of the upper and lower anatomical bounds outside of which a theory of brain function must not venture.

First, let us consider Mountcastle's own estimates. He starts with the assumption that the total neocortical volume of the human brain is about 1,000 cm^3, and the mean cortical thickness is 2,500 μm. This implies a neocortical surface area of 4,000 cm^2, which implies 567 million minicolumns (30 μm diameter) over the entire brain, or 283 million per cerebral hemisphere.

Other published estimates of the total cortical surface area, however, are substantially lower than Mountcastle's 4,000 cm^2 estimate (2,000 cm^2 per hemisphere) – suggesting that Mountcastle's starting assumption of a neocortical volume of 1,000 cm^3 (which Mountcastle makes no attempt at justifying in what was admittedly an order of magnitude estimate) may be exaggerated. Empirically the volume of the cerebral cortex has been reported at least four times: those values are 230.4, 310, 510 and 566 cm^3. This 2.5-fold difference between the smallest and largest values is disturbing, but undoubtedly our best estimate will lie somewhere below Mountcastle's estimate of 1,000 cm^3.

Based upon evolutionary and phylogenetic considerations, Hofman (1983) has calculated a total cortical surface area of 3,076 cm^2 (1,538 cm^2 per hemisphere). In 1910 Henneberg reported a figure of 1,090 cm^2 as the mean of seven normal human cerebral hemispheres using a laborious technique of spreading gold foil over the entire brain surface. More recently Elias and Schwartz (1969) reported a similar figure (2,275 cm^2 for the entire cortex or 1,137.5 cm^2 per hemisphere), using an empirical stereological method. The close agreement between those two empirical values is noteworthy, and the discrepancy with theoretical values can be understood as follows. If we correct for shrinkage of 18 percent in each linear direction (Rockel et al., 1980) due to formalin fixation, then the Henneberg areal value can be corrected to 1,602 cm^2 and the Elias and Schwartz value to 1,692 cm^2, that is in rough agreement with Hofman's theoretical value (1,538 cm^2), although still considerably smaller than Mountcastle's estimate of 2,000 cm^2 per hemisphere.

It should be noted that the corrected empirical values obtained by Henneberg and by Elias and Schwartz are similar to those of seven other pre-1950 values for the cortical surface area of non-fixated cerebral hemispheres, as obtained by various groups and reported in Blinkov and Glezer (1968); they are 1,497 cm^2, 1,560 cm^2, 1,600 cm^2, 1,610 cm^2, 1,622 cm^2, 1,635 cm^2, and 1,671 cm^2 (mean = 1,599 cm^2). Particularly noteworthy is Weil's (1928, cited in Blinkov and Glezer, 1968) study of the effects of formalin fixation. The pre-fixation value was 1,622 cm^2, whereas the post-fixation value was $1,438$ cm^2 (implying a linear shrinkage of 9.4 percent in both dimensions of the cortical surface). Due to the natural variation of brain sizes among normal individuals, a more precise estimate may not be possible. Suffice it to say that our best estimate of the area of the cortex of one normal, human cerebral hemisphere is between $1,500$ and $1,700$ cm^2.

The inexactitude of each of the figures under consideration makes firm conclusions impossible, but the importance of obtaining a first approximation should be emphasized. That is if it were found that the number of cortical units is orders of magnitude larger than the number of callosal fibers, then the role of the corpus callosum could not possibly be a point-to-point topographical representation of information from one hemisphere to the other. In such a case a gross 'activation' or 'suppression' of the contralateral hemisphere might be possible, but a gross disparity between the number of cortical columns and the number of connecting fibers would make topographical mapping, such as found in the visual pathway, unlikely.

The calculations above suggest that the number of cortical columns in a cerebral hemisphere could not exceed 234 million. Most estimates of the number of neurons in the cerebral cortex have been between 5 and 10 billion (table 222, Blinkov and Glezer, 1968) – a range which would imply only 50–100 million minicolumns per hemisphere. The accuracy of such estimates is uncertain, but if they are justifiable, then already there are few enough minicolumns that two or more callosal fibers could connect all homologous columns between the hemispheres. While the corpus callosum in man may in fact contain as many as 200 million fibers, it should be noted that a topographical mapping theory of callosal function (excitatory or inhibitory) requires *two* callosal fibers for each pair of homologous cortical columns, such that mutual inhibition or excitation could occur. Unless, therefore, the 200–250 million fiber estimate of the human corpus callosum is a gross underestimation, it appears unlikely that a topographical theory of callosal function can be built upon the minimal anatomical unit of the cortex, Mountcastle's minicolumn (diameter $= 30$ μm). Nevertheless the crucial questions about callosal function are concerned not with the anatomical minicolumns, but with the interhemispheric relations of the homologous functional units, i.e. Mountcastle's macrocolumns.

Since, outside of striate cortex, all functional macrocolumns are larger than the minimum anatomical unit), estimates of the numbers of functional macrocolumns per hemisphere will necessarily be smaller than the maximum minicolumn estimate of 234 million. If 250 million is indeed our best estimate of the number of callosal fibers, then one-half that figure or 125 million for the number of macrocolumns is the crucial upper limit which a topographical mapping theory of the corpus callosum can withstand. Only if there are twice as many callosal fibers as functional units in each cerebral hemisphere could mutual effects by

Table 2.2 Areal measures of brain regions

Region of brain[1] (see figure A1.1)	Mean and s.d. of seven hemispheres[2] (sq. mm)	Percentage of cortex (range)	Filiminov (1949)	Glezer (1963)
Frontal I	10,281±1,697	9.5		
Frontal II	8,347±744	7.7		
Frontal III	5,035±796	4.7		
Basal frontal lobe	7,268±1,090	6.7		
Precentral gyrus	6,817±367	6.3		
Total frontal lobe	37,749±2,775	35.0 (33.6–37.4%)	32.8	34.0
Temporal I	6,306±521	5.9		
Temporal II	12,956±1,827	12.0		
Total temporal	19,262±1,835	17.9 (16.8–18.8%)	23.5	23.4[5]
Postcentral gyrus	5,006±825	4.6		
Parietal lobe	16,960±1,524	15.7		
Total parietal lobe	21,966±2,157	20.4 (18.6–22.0%)	21.5	16.9[5]

Total occipital lobe	17,199 ± 1,791	15.7 (13.9–17.5%)	12.0	13.0
Cingulate gyrus	6,806 ± 1,042	6.0		
Uncal gyrus	2,521 ± 339	2.5		
Total limbic lobe	9,327 ± 1,381	8.5 (7.4–10.5%)	8.4[3]	10.6[4]
Insula	2,218 ± 206	2.1 (1.7–2.4%)	1.8	2.1
Total cortex	107,721 ± 7,644	100%	100%	100%

Notes: 1. brain regions as defined by Henneberg (1910) (see figure 2.22). 2. from Henneberg (1910). 3. calculated as the sum of all non-neocortical regions plus 4.0% 'limbic cortex' from table 183 of Blinkov and Glezer (1968). 4. calculated as the remainder of unaccounted-for cortex in table 190 of Blinkov and Glezer (1968). 5. the discrepancy between the Henneberg and the Filiminov and Glezer values for total temporal and occipital lobe areas is most likely due to differences in the status of the lingual and fusiform gyri. Both of these gyri are part temporal and part occipital with no obvious anatomical demarcation to define them (see appendix 1 and figure A1.2).

homologous units occur and therefore allow for the possibility of inhibitory or excitatory topographical mapping.

Consequently by calculating the number of cortical macrocolumns over each area of cortex from the known macrocolumn diameters and from the known relative areas of various cortical regions, estimates can be obtained of the total number of functional units.

Table 2.2 shows the relative and absolute areal measures of the major subdivisions of the cortex, based upon the empirical values of Henneberg (1910). The boundaries of the various cortical subregions used by Henneberg are summarized in figure 2.22. Also shown in table 2.2 are the percentage values of the cortical lobes obtained by Filiminov (1949, cited in Blinkov and Glezer, 1968) and Glezer *et al.* (1963, cited in Blinkov and Glezer, 1968). Using the percentage values reported by Henneberg and the known sizes of the macrocolumns in various cortical areas, total hemispheric macrocolumn estimates can be made. First, the surface areas of the major cortical regions were calculated (based upon the total cortical areas obtained empirically by Henneberg, 1910, and Elias and Schwartz, 1969, and theoretically by Hofman, 1983). These values are summarized in table 2.3.

Finally, using the areal measures listed in table 2.3, the number of

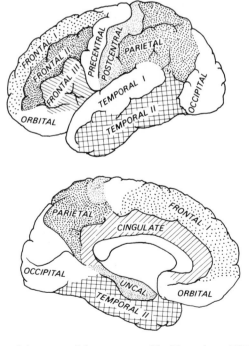

Figure 2.22 The subdivisions of the cortex used by Henneberg (1910) in his measurements of various cortical regions (see tables 2.2–2.4).

Table 2.3 Estimates of the size of various cortical regions

Cortical region[1]	Percentage of cortex	Area[2] (sq. cm)	Area[3] (sq. cm)	Area[4] (sq. cm)
Frontal I	9.5	160.7	152.2	146.1
Frontal II	7.7	130.3	123.4	118.4
Frontal III	4.7	79.5	75.3	72.3
Frontal basal	6.7	113.4	107.3	103.0
Precentral gyrus	6.3	106.6	100.9	96.9
Total frontal lobe	35.0	592.2	560.7	538.3
Parietal I	4.6	77.8	73.7	70.7
Parietal II	15.7	265.6	251.5	241.5
Total parietal lobe	20.4	345.2	326.8	313.8
Temporal I	5.9	99.8	94.5	90.7
Temporal II	12.0	203.0	192.2	184.6
Total temporal lobe	17.9	302.9	286.8	275.3
Total occipital lobe	15.7	265.6	251.5	241.5
Total insular cortex	2.1	35.5	33.6	32.3
Uncal gyrus	2.3	38.9	36.8	35.4
Cingulate cyrus	6.3	106.6	100.9	96.9
Total limbic lobe	8.7	147.2	139.4	133.8
Total cortex	100	1,692	1,602	1,538

Notes: 1. percentages calculated from the mean areal measures of seven hemispheres given by Henneberg (1910) (see figure 2.22). 2. based upon a corrected (18% enlargement in both dimensions of the cortical surface) value of 1,692 sq. cm for the hemispheric surface obtained by Elias and Schwartz (1969). 3. based upon a similarly corrected value of 1,602 sq. cm for the cortical surface area obtained by Henneberg (1910). 4. based upon Hofman's (1983) (uncorrected) estimate of 1,538 sq. cm obtained by means of evolutionary considerations.

cortical columns which could be squeezed into each cortical region can be calculated from the known size of cortical columns in the various cortical regions (see table 2.4). All assumptions required for the calculations listed in the tables are made to maximize the total number of cortical columns. For example, the macrocolumn diameter in striate cortex is said to be 30 μm, so this dimension is assumed for all of visual cortex (Brodmann's areas 17, 18 and 19). Similarly dimensions of 50 μm and 200 μm are the minimal macrocolumn diameters in auditory and somatosensory cortex, so calculations have been made assuming those dimensions for the respective regions of primary sensory cortex. Such assumptions provide us with maximum macrocolumn estimates,

Table 2.4 Estimates of the number of cortical macrocolumns in each cerebral hemisphere

Cortical region[1] (% of total cortex)	Diameter of macrocolumn	Number of macrocolumns[2]	Number of macrocolumns[3]	Number of macrocolumns[4]
Visual cortex (15.7%)	30 μm	34,160,400	37,580,900	44,421,900
Auditory cortex (5.9%)	50 μm	4,621,450	5,084,200	6,009,690
Somesthetic cortex (4.6%)	200 μm	225,198	247,747	292,845
Motor cortex (6.3%)	500 μm	49,348	54,289	64,171
All other cortical regions (67.5%)				
Assumption (i)	30 μm	146,868,000	161,574,000	190,986,000
Assumption (ii)	50 μm	52,872,600	58,166,700	68,755,000
Assumption (iii)	100 μm	13,218,100	14,541,700	17,188,700
Assumption (iv)	200 μm	3,304,530	3,635,420	4,297,180

Total numbers of cortical columns

(i) Under the assumption that the macrocolumn diameter in 'all other regions' is 30 μm	Mean macrocolumn diameter of 69 μm	185,924,396	204,541,136	241,774,606

(ii) Under the assumption that the macrocolumn diameter in 'all other regions' is 50 μm	Mean macrocolumn diameter of 82 μm	91,928,996	101,133,836	119,543,606
(iii) Under the assumption that the macrocolumn diameter in 'all other regions' is 100 μm	Mean macrocolumn diameter of 116 μm	53,274,496	57,508,436	67,977,306
(iv) Under the assumption that the macrocolumn diameter in 'all other regions' is 200 μm	Mean macrocolumn diameter of 183 μm	42,360,926	46,602,556	55,085,786

Notes: 1. percentage values from Henneberg (1910). 2. based upon Hofman's (1983) estimate of the hemispherical surface area of 1,538 sq. cm. 3. based upon a corrected value of 1,692 sq. cm after Elias and Schwartz (1969). 4. based upon Mountcastle's (1978) estimate of a hemispherical surface area of 2,000 sq. cm.

which are consequently the most conservative figures for a topographical mapping theory of the corpus callosum. As can be seen from the lower half of table 2.4, all estimates of the number of macrocolumns in a cerebral hemisphere are less than 125 million, except the estimates based upon the assumption that all cortical columns of frontal, parietal and temporal 'association' areas have diameters approximately equal to those of visual striate cortex (= 30 μm). All other combinations of assumptions produce figures of fewer than 125 million cortical columns per cerebral hemisphere – i.e. less than one-half the number of callosal fibers. It is therefore concluded that there is a sufficient number of callosal fibers relative to the number of functional units of the cortex to allow for topographical transferral of information from one hemisphere to the other.

An important question remains concerning the termination of callosal fibers. If individual neurons of the corpus callosum send axons to a relatively widespread region of the contralateral cortex (region of termination $>>$ functional units), then it is questionable whether or not topographical specificity could be maintained. If, on the other hand, there is specificity of termination which is comparable to the size of the cortical macrocolumns, then there are grounds for defending a topographical theory of callosal function.

It is worth noting, however, that – despite considerable changes in the numbers of elements at various stages in visual processing – topographical mapping is maintained at least as far as striate cortex. Specifically, although the retina is known to have approximately 126 million rods and cones, the optic tract carries all of its information along a tract of only 3 million fibers. At striate cortex, this information is again expanded over a cortical region estimate to have upwards of 20 million cortical columns. A deficiency in the number of callosal fibers relative to cortical columns might not, therefore, be a fatal blow to a topographical theory of callosal function, but some indication of mechanisms of 'convergence' would certainly need to be demonstrated.

Empirical findings concerning this question are unambiguous. Wolf and Zaborsky (1979) found that: '(1) columns are often delimited from each other by narrow rims containing fewer callosal terminals than the centers, and (2) within columns the highly variable laminar distribution pattern of callosal terminals is uniform, but may change from one column to another; this has become a good criterion for delimiting columns.' 'Using these criteria, the columns form cylinders with an average diameter of 150–250 μm extending through the whole thickness of the cortex. . . . Wider columns (diameter: 350–500 μm) can be identified mostly by one of the above-mentioned criteria, as complex columns being composed of several fused columnar units.' Those findings were obtained in the rat neocortex (including areas 18, 39, 40, 1, 2 and 3), but comparable results have been obtained by Goldman and

Nauta (1977) and Jones *et al.* (1975) with regard to corticocortical fibers in monkeys (see figure 2.23).

Since the corpus callosum is but one variety of corticocortical fiber, 'the similar diameter in monkeys and rats [about 200 μm], the common tendency to fuse, forming complex columns, patches, bands, etc., as well as the presence of 'empty columns,' might indicate that columns represent a more general unit of space organization in the cortex' (Wolff and Zaborsky, 1979). Similarly Hedreen and Yin (1981) note:

> Though relatively few insights into commissural functions have yet emerged, the corpus callosum nevertheless furnishes a striking example of the precision of connections that can be found in the nervous system. Within the connected regions, callosal fibers terminate in a pronounced columnar fashion that resembles the well-known ocular dominance columns.

In *Architectonics of the Cerebral Cortex* Szentagothai (1978b) states that:

> Although there is virtually no possibility anatomically for anything like a point-to-point connectivity on the level of single cells in long-

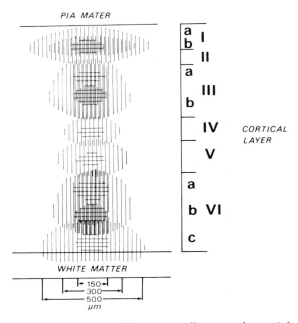

Figure 2.23 Laminar termination of the corpus callosum in the rat (after Wolff and Zaborsky, 1979). The horizontal lines indicate the center of the callosal terminations, and the vertical lines the spread or scatter of termination. The cortical column is found to be a 'corsetted cylinder.' In the monkey, chimpanzee and probably man, there is no termination of callosal fibers in layers I and II; rather, the highest density of termination is in layer IV, but some termination in layers III, V and VI is also found.

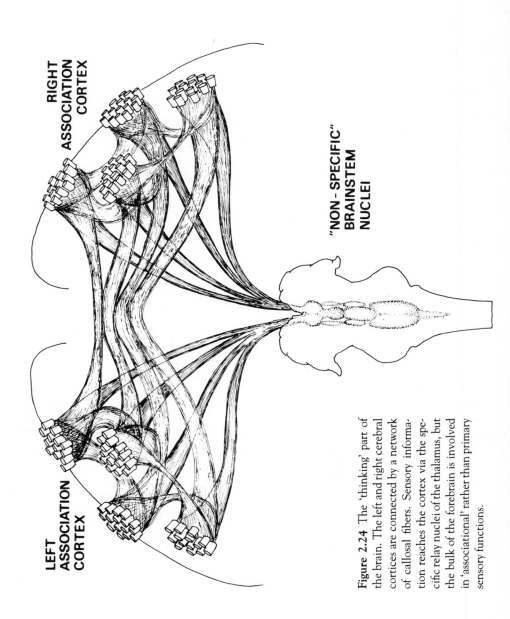

LEFT ASSOCIATION CORTEX

RIGHT ASSOCIATION CORTEX

"NON - SPECIFIC" BRAINSTEM NUCLEI

Figure 2.24 The 'thinking' part of the brain. The left and right cerebral cortices are connected by a network of callosal fibers. Sensory information reaches the cortex via the specific relay nuclei of the thalamus, but the bulk of the forebrain is involved in 'associational' rather than primary sensory functions.

and medium-range connexions, such a predetermined specificity can be realistically assumed for relatively small pieces (columns) of cortex with cell numbers within the order of magnitude of 100.

In conclusion, the anatomical evidence concerning the number of callosal fibers and the number of cortical columns indicate that there are enough fibers to allow the *functional macrocolumns* of large portions of the cortex of one hemisphere – perhaps the entire expanse of neocortex which is neither primary sensory nor primary motor cortex – to send and receive two or more callosal fibers. This approximate ratio of two callosal fibers for every one cortical column implies that a *topographical* relationship between the hemispheres is anatomically possible. Our next question therefore becomes: Is the topographical relationship between the cerebral hemispheres across the corpus callosum excitatory or inhibitory?

Summary

The brain can be conveniently dissected into three principal functional units: the centrally located brainstem, which is involved in the activation and inhibition of limited portions of the cortex; the cortex itself, which is divided into two 1,600 cm^2 sheets containing a multitude of two-dimensional representations of sensory and motor information; and the corpus callosum, which forms a bridge between the two cortical sheets and allows them to communicate (figure 2.24).

The current trend in research on the functions of the neocortex is toward finding more and more two-dimensional representations of the motor and sensory fields – generally accurate, if somewhat distorted reconstructions of the external world. There is a proportional decrease in the amount of cortex which can be labeled 'associational' – and these areas which are known to be multimodal are likely to be regions containing 'overlapping maps' from different sense organs.

The nature of the communication among these maps along cortico-cortical fibers remains uncertain, but a large percentage of the so-called white matter of the brain is devoted specifically to that task. The largest single tract of this kind is the corpus callosum. Elucidation of its mechanisms of action would undoubtedly throw light on hemispheric relations (lateral specializations and dominance), in particular, and corticocortical communication, in general.

3

FUNCTIONS OF THE CORPUS CALLOSUM

Historically functions of an extreme nature have been attributed to the corpus callosum. From its massive size and central location, early philosophers concluded that it was 'the seat of the soul' (Gordon, 1974), yet in the first half of the twentieth century no functions of any kind could be identified by most neurosurgeons and even its usefulness as a nerve tract was questioned. Since the start of the 'split-brain' studies, there has been a small return of respectability for this nerve tract – but it is probably fair to say that current ideas of callosal function have been more heavily influenced by the negative conclusions of the 1930s and 1940s than by the philosophical considerations of previous centuries. It is now recognized that the forebrain commissures do have functions, but not functions of such a central and crucial importance that we can attribute metaphysical properties to them.

More than anything else, research on men and animals which have undergone transection of the corpus callosum has shown that sensory information received in one hemisphere is normally shunted across to the other side when the callosum is intact, but not so after a longitudinal cut through the brain. The importance of letting the other half of the nervous system know what is going on contralaterally may be self-evident, but clearly the distribution of sensory information must be described as a lower-level function. In the auditory modality, callosal connections are thought to play a role in the localization of a sound source relative to the midline of the head and, particularly in vision (where there is relatively little direct input to each hemisphere of ipsilateral visual information), the corpus callosum is probably essential for unifying the sensory field. Few researchers, however, would today assert that the corpus callosum plays an important role in consciousness.

There have nonetheless been sporadic indications from both clinical and experimental studies that the functions of the corpus callosum transcend the narrow interests of the sensory physiologist. While unification of the sensory field may in fact be one important role, many have speculated about callosal functions other than the distribution of sensory information.

In a history of thought on the corpus callosum, Bogen (1979) has identified five stages, labeled as follows: (i) the humoral anatomists, (ii) the traffic anatomists, (iii) the classical neurologists, (iv) their critics, and (v) the two-brain theorists. To this sequence I would add a sixth stage, the integrationists.

The humoral anatomists included various natural philosophers who were more impressed with the cerebrospinal fluid and its brain cavities than with the substance of the brain itself. They considered the central location of the corpus callosum to be important – primarily as a support structure which allowed the brain liquor to slosh around in enlightening ways. More than 100 years later, the traffic anatomists (Willis, Descartes and others) realized the importance of the solid matter of the brain, and were also struck by various midline structures, notably the pineal gland and the corpus callosum. If the brain is where our thoughts come from, then certainly our best thoughts must come from the center of our brains!

Following after these early natural philosophers, but borrowing few of their ideas, the classical neurologists through the 1930s settled down to record the signs and symptoms of callosal disease and to build the foundations of the terminology and content of modern neurology. One of the many debates which they initiated was whether or not tumors, transection or agenesis of the corpus callosum produce notable behavioral or psychic symptoms. The idea of unilateral left-sided dominance for language functions became established during this period, but the identification of a 'callosal syndrome' did not survive the harsh remarks of 'the critics.'

Despite many clinical cases showing psychological and behavioral deficits associated with callosal disorders, the idea of a specific 'syndrome' was disputed. Mental symptoms were not always evident and were often difficult to specify with precision. Suggestions of 'apathy,' 'difficulties in concentration' and 'bizarreness of manner' were easily ridiculed as unscientific by the critics of the callosal syndrome, and the more concrete behavioral disorders of the callosal syndrome (agraphia, unilateral neglect, etc.) were sometimes not found and usually subsided rapidly. Finally early animal experiments failed to reveal any significant deficits following callosal section – again reducing the corpus callosum (in the eyes of the critics) to merely a support structure!

Not until the 1960s was anything approaching agreement on at least some callosal functions achieved. It was then found that, given the appropriate testing conditions, considerable independence of the cerebral hemispheres could be demonstrated following callosal transection in both man and animals. This empirical fact led some psychologists to the extreme view that the corpus callosum connects two relatively independent brains and therefore perhaps two more-or-less autonomous minds (see, for example, Ornstein, 1972). Particularly in light of some of the bizarre anecdotes concerning the split-brain patients, it was perhaps inevitable that the 'two brains' and even the 'two personalities inside one skull' viewpoint would be taken to its Californian limit. Although the reevaluation of the human nervous system in terms of its

77

fundamental bilaterality was undoubtedly an important return to fundamental issues, the extremes of the two-brain viewpoint have more recently led to another swing of the pendulum to a more unitary view of the functions of the central nervous system, the integrationist perspective.

Although it could be said that the two-brain perspective implicitly recognizes the importance of the corpus callosum in normally joining the cerebral hemispheres, the emphasis in 'two-brain theory' has been not on what this nerve tract does, but on what it hides. Rather than focusing on the active role of the connecting fibers, the two-brain position focuses on the *separate* specializations of the hemispheres – especially when the two 'brains' have been surgically separated or tricked by experimental techniques into separate and contradictory functioning.

Certainly the empirical basis for the two-brain theory has never been stronger and is convincingly in evidence in some of the dramatically self-contradictory split-brain subjects, but a dissatisfaction with the Dr Jekyll and Mr Hyde characterization of the human brain, together with a renewed interest in the integrating and coordinating aspects of the corpus callosum, has led to a sixth stage of thought concerning callosal functions, that of the integrationists. It might be argued that the integrationist perspective is nothing more than one school of thought within the two-brain theory, if for no other reason than that many of the experimental techniques and clinical findings are the same as those used by the two-brain theorists, but the emphasis on the nature of brain functions has certainly changed. Instead of asking how different the two sides of the brain can be, the integrationists have asked how the corpus callosum normally combines those differences into a unified whole. Representative of the integrationist perspective are Gazzaniga and LeDoux (1978) and Kinsbourne (1978, 1982).

The main purpose of this and the following chapter is therefore to outline the integrationist perspective in its various forms and to argue the case for considering the corpus callosum as having a significant role in human cognition. Let it be said that modern anatomy and physiology indicate that the corpus callosum is very much like all other corticocortical fibers. Because of its large size, midline location and rapid evolutionary development, its importance, as compared to other association fibers, may be enhanced, but we are not in a position to speculate about the soulfulness or spiritual properties of this or any other nerve tract. At best, we might be able to show that the corpus callosum plays a role in normal thought processes, but we must leave questions of consciousness and the soul to be answered by philosophers and metaphysicians.

The importance of understanding the corpus callosum may be evident already from its size and position alone, but there is another, related factor which emphasizes its importance to experimental psychology: because the corpus callosum traverses the gap between the hemispheres, it can be approached experimentally more easily than other association fibers. It is therefore not only a tract of great theoretical interest since it joins the two 'brains,' but also one of the most easily manipulated portions of the central nervous system and the *only* corticocortical tract which can be manipulated without doing damage to the cortex itself. So if there remain secrets concerning how information is transferred from one region of cortex to another, the corpus callosum stands the best chance of revealing the mechanisms involved.

Not surprisingly, two of the leading researchers on the split-brain patients, Sperry and Gazzaniga, clearly feel that elucidation of callosal functions is a crucial step in deciphering the brain code. Sperry (1974) has noted:

> More than any other cerebral system, the interhemispheric commissures and their cortical associations continue to offer promise in the search for an eventual direct correlation between the phenomena of complex subjective experience and known variables in specified neural structures.

Gazzaniga has stated in *The Bisected Brain* (1970):

> Since the corpus callosum is the only fiber tract in the brain that we know transmits high-order information, . . . any clarification of its processing logic would be of enormous value in attaining clues on the larger questions of the brain code.

It is therefore disconcerting how little has been published explicitly on the corpus callosum (although the lack of clinical implications is the likely cause). Only three previous books have appeared in English over the past twenty years: *Functions of the Corpus Callosum* (edited by Ettlinger, 1965), *Structure and Function of the Cerebral Commissures* (edited by Russell *et al.*, 1979), and *Epilepsy and the Corpus Callosum* (edited by Reeves, 1985). Still the amount of experimental, theoretical and philosophical material relevant to callosal functions is stupendous if we consider the sum total of work done on brain laterality and hemispheric specialization. Noteworthy among the books which are not edited collections of research papers are: *The Bisected Brain* (Gazzaniga, 1970), *The Double Brain* (Dimond, 1972), *The Psychology of Left and Right* (Corballis and Beale, 1976), *The Integrated Mind* (Gazzaniga and LeDoux, 1978), *Human Cerebral Asymmetry* (Bradshaw and Nettleton, 1983) and *Cerebral Basis of Psychopathology* (Flor-Henry, 1983). These books on hemisphere function and dysfunction provide the essential background material for considerations of callosal functions, but the interested reader will find a curious paucity of discussion of the corpus callosum in all of them!

Current ideas concerning callosal function

In modern times virtually all hypotheses concerning the functions of the corpus callosum have been within the framework of either 'two-brain' or 'integrationist' theory. Regardless of which perspective they would support, such hypotheses have emphasized either the primarily excitatory or the primarily inhibitory nature of this fiber tract. They have also differed fundamentally with regard to the specificity of the presumed callosal effects – the cerebral hemispheres either having effects on one another which increase or decrease their levels of general activity (diffuse effects) or having effects which allow for the transmission of cortical 'information' (topographical effects). There are consequently four general classes of callosal hypothesis (table 3.1) – each of which has been defended in recent years.

THE TOPOGRAPHICAL EXCITATORY HYPOTHESIS

The topographical excitatory or 'carbon-copy' hypothesis was first suggested by Sperry (1962) and since developed by Berlucchi (1981, 1983), but it has been the implicit theory behind many discussions of callosal functions. In this hypothesis, approximate bilateral symmetry of the cerebral hemispheres and predominantly homotopic callosal connections between columnar units of the cortex are assumed. In other words, mirror-image patches of cortex on the left and right are

Table 3.1 A summary of callosal hypotheses

	Net excitatory effects	Net inhibitory effects
Topographical effects of callosal fibers (as a consequence, the configuration of callosal termination is informational)	Sperry (1962) Gazzaniga (1970) Gazzaniga and LeDoux (1978) Berlucchi (1983)	Kinsbourne (1974, 1982) Doty *et al.* (1973, 1977, 1979) Cook (1984a, b, c)
Diffuse effects of callosal fibers (as a consequence, the configuration of callosal termination is non-informational, i.e. modulating contralateral arousal)	Guiard (1980)	Dimond (1977) Galin (1977) Denenberg (1980, 1981, 1983)

connected by callosal fibers, whose net effect is to convey the information on one side to the other.

Provided that the 'point-to-point' specificity of callosal fibers is between cortical columns (diameter > 50 μm) rather than between individual neurons, i.e. no more precise than the degree of specificity probable for medium- and long-range fibers (Szentagothai, 1978a), then the calculations on pp. 58–72 show that there are more than enough callosal fibers to connect all such homotopic columns at least twice. Since our best estimate of the neocortical surface area in one human cerebral hemisphere is approximately 1,600 cm^2, it could contain about 100 million cortical columns (with a mean diameter of 100–200 μm) and therefore allow for two callosal fibers between every pair of homotopic cortical columns.

It therefore appears that the specificity required in the topographical excitatory callosal hypothesis is well within the constraints which are imposed by the total hemispheric surface area and estimates concerning the number of callosal fibers. With regard to the physiological effects of callosal activity, animal studies have shown that stimulation of the cerebral cortex in one hemisphere or callosal fibers results in brief excitation followed by prolonged inhibition in the contralateral homotopic region (see p. 101). Although such findings are often considered as support for the 'traditional' inhibitory view of callosal function, the reality of both excitatory and inhibitory effects makes it possible that this commissure allows for the excitatory topographical transfer of a pattern of cortical activity to the contralateral hemisphere. Particularly in primary sensory cortical regions, the precise point-to-point transfer of information may be important in the production of a unified sensory field (Sperry, 1962) and essential for stereopsis (Mitchell and Blakemore, 1970) (see chapter 6).

It is of interest in this regard that, although attributable to Sperry, the excitatory topographical theory of callosal function was not further developed by him. Experimentally he and others have demonstrated the 'transfer of information' from one hemisphere to the other in numerous animal studies, but comments on the nature of the transfer and the neuronal mechanisms involved have usually been omitted from the discussion of experimental results. Sperry himself (1962) noted that excitatory homotopic callosal connections 'would appear to be about as helpful as a double exposure in photography.' Insofar as the retinotopic 'maps' on homotopic cortical regions are *not* mirror-images of one another, but contain differing information concerning primarily the contralateral hemifield, homotopic callosal connections would appear to serve no useful function. It has since been found that in fact much of *primary* sensory cortex does not have callosal fibers, so that homotopic callosal excitation at other regions remains a strong theoretical candidate.

One important implication of the excitatory model should be noted.

It relies heavily on anatomical asymmetries of the cerebral hemispheres to explain functional asymmetries and, moreover, it implies a correspondingly small number of anatomical asymmetries elsewhere in the animal kingdom where laterality effects are much smaller. A related implication of the excitatory model is that all functional asymmetries are due to inherent differences between the hemispheres and *not* due to callosal activity. Weiskrantz (1979, 1980) has argued that the very fact of such numerous interhemispheric fibers implies that the cerebral hemispheres must contain different information which needs to be transferred to the other side. Why else would mammalian brains bother with such a massive network of fibers? It is in fact the case that the hemispheres receive somewhat different sensory information from the separate sensory half-fields, but it is worth pointing out that all callosal functions need not be excitatory. Either inhibition as a means of producing 'dominance' (the diffuse inhibitory hypothesis, described on pp. 82–7) or inhibitory information transfer (the topographical inhibitory model, described on pp. 88–91) would be mechanisms by which different kinds of information could be *produced* by callosal activity. It does not therefore follow that the mere presence of commissural fibers indicates preexisting hemispheric asymmetries which the callosal 'telephone exchange' will then relay to the other side.

It remains to be seen how close a correlation between anatomical (gross morphological, cytoarchitectonic or neurotransmitter) asymmetries and functional asymmetries will eventually be demonstrated in man and other animal species, but the excitatory theories demand a very high correlation insofar as no additional callosal mechanism can be invoked. In fairness, whether or not reduction to the cellular level will work in the case of brain lateralization remains uncertain, but at least one question will need to be given a satisfactory answer within the excitatory model before the reductionist argument can be taken seriously: How does the corpus callosum function? If there exist two 'cortical modules' specialized for, say, musical chord recognition on the right and phonemic analysis on the left, how does callosal activity allow for meaningful communication between them and why should it bother? Why, moreover, are callosal connections homotopic? And why is there such a massive phylogenetic increase in the number of callosal fibers?

THE DIFFUSE INHIBITORY HYPOTHESIS

Undoubtedly the difficulties posed by such questions have led to the relative popularity among psychologists of an inhibitory view of callosal functions. Again, assuming some degree of hemispheric specialization due to the inherent structural asymmetries, an inhibitory corpus callosum would allow one cortical region to be active while its contralateral homolog would be suppressed. If psychological functions are localized to various cortical regions (lobes, lobules, gyri or other macroscopic but well-defined areas), then a cerebral hemisphere could establish virtually complete dominance by means of contralateral inhibition. This is the essence of the widely held, but infrequently examined, diffuse inhibitory callosal model.

Despite the apparent simplicity of a topographical excitatory model in which a pattern of cortical activity is transmitted in its entirety to the other hemisphere, it has in fact been the case that most previous hypotheses concerning callosal functions (especially those concerned with the role of the corpus callosum in corticocortical communications between association areas) have been based upon predominantly *inhibitory* effects. Diffuse callosal inhibition has been invoked to account for normal laterality effects in man – that is the fact that there is handedness and language dominance in most people *despite* massive interhemispheric communications (e.g. Corballis and Morgan, 1978). Inhibition has also been invoked to explain the postoperative changes in the split-brain patients – generally an increase in the similarity of the cerebral hemispheres over time, as if the differentiating influences of the corpus callosum had been removed (e.g. Moscovitch, 1976). Moreover, it has been argued that a loss of inhibition is behind the cognitive abnormalities of individuals with callosal agenesis (e.g. Dennis, 1976). Even the laterality findings in sub-human species seem to find their easiest explanation in terms of a normally inhibitory functioning of the forebrain commissures (e.g. Denenberg, 1980, 1981). Finally it is noteworthy that thus far all hypotheses designed to account for the abnormalities of hemispheric dominance in psychopathological states have been based upon a *normally inhibitory* role of the corpus callosum and an *abnormally excitatory* role (manifest in conditions such as epilepsy and schizophrenia) (e.g. Flor-Henry, 1983; Wexler and Heninger, 1979). The relative popularity of inhibitory models among psychologists is evident.

It should be noted, however, that most of these ideas concerning the corpus callosum are actually concerned with the 'net effect' of interhemispheric communications rather than the physiology of the corpus callosum itself. Since the inhibitory phase of cortical activity, due to callosal firing, follows a short excitatory burst (see pp. 101–2), it is generally thought that callosal effects are inhibitory only after having passed through an appropriate inhibitory interneuron. In other words, the callosal fibers themselves may indeed have excitatory effects on contralateral interneurons and the debate concerning callosal functions may really be concerned with subsequent effects. To the physiologist this is a crucial distinction, but to the psychologist the final outcome of the neuronal processes is of central importance. Strictly speaking both views may be correct – the corpus callosum having monosynaptically excitatory effects and disynaptically inhibitory effects, but the nature of the information transferred should differ radically depending upon which process predominates.

One of the principal attractions of the diffuse inhibitory view of the corpus callosum is that it allows for the possibility of asymmetric hemisphere function without resorting to additional assumptions concerning the inherent asymmetry of the brain. To be sure, some such asymmetries are known, but it is simply not clear what kinds of anatomical or physiological asymmetries could produce functional asymmetries. Whereas an excitatory model of callosal function implies that activity of the corpus callosum *reduces* hemispheric specializations due to 'cross-talk,' an inhibitory model implies that the specializations themselves are due at least partially to callosal effects (and as such no recourse to lower-level asymmetries are needed). In this sense the excitatory theory is implicitly a reductionist argument concerning brain laterality, whereas the inhibitory theory is implicitly a systems theoretical argument. Both perspectives, we shall find, have their separate realms of validity.

These contrasting implications of the diffuse inhibitory and topographical excitatory theories of callosal function are rarely commented on, but they are important for the development of a theoretical understanding of cerebral laterality effects. The fact that excitatory callosal effects would tend to bring the cerebral hemispheres toward greater symmetry of activity clearly indicates that, if indeed this tract is predominantly excitatory, then hemispheric functional *asymmetries* must be due to structural and functional mechanisms other than those of the corpus callosum itself. Gross morphological and cytoarchitectonic differences between the hemispheres are the obvious place to begin the search for other 'lateralizing' mechanisms, but the implied tendency toward 'bilateralization' of function – from which the excitatory theory cannot escape – must be dealt with somewhere within the excitatory model. In other words, if the corpus callosum is predominantly excitatory, the greater its activity, the greater must be the similarity between the cerebral hemispheres.

In contrast the inhibitory theories of callosal function imply hemispheric asymmetries due at least partially to the activity of this fiber tract. If, for whatever reason, one hemisphere were transiently to become 'dominant' for a given function, its capacity to inhibit the contralateral hemisphere would inevitably further augment that 'dominance.' Unlike an excitatory effect, inhibition would have an inherent 'lateralizing' effect – increasing the differences in electrical activity and presumably the informational content of the two hemispheres.

The diffuse inhibitory models have suffered, however, from a lack of plausible physiology. Galin (1977), Dimond (1977) and others have suggested that there is a rather diffuse inhibition of large contralateral cortical regions – for example, inhibition of the right-sided homolog of Broca's area during left-sided verbal activity. Corballis and Morgan (1978) have argued for developmental suppression of the right hemisphere by the left during fetal development and Ornstein (1972) has suggested that there might be a rapid switching between the cerebral hemispheres, with concomitant alternating modes of thought. It is unclear, however, how such inhibition, suppression or switching might work and this lack of physiological detail has prevented the diffuse inhibitory model from extending beyond the realm of the 'conceptual nervous system.'

The weaknesses of this view have recently been brought into focus in an exchange between Denenberg and Berlucchi. In response to Denenberg's contention (1981) that mutual inhibition may be one important mechanism inducing hemispheric specializations in man and animals, Berlucchi (1983) argued that such an inhibitory relationship should result in, but empirically is not found to result in, large hemispheric asymmetries using physiological measures of brain activity, regional cerebral blood flow (rCBF) and glucose metabolism. Berlucchi concluded that the *functional unit* of the brain is likely to be pairs of homologous cortical columns in the left and right hemispheres with *excitatory* callosal connections. Such cortical columns would be activated in approximate unison due to callosal effects, resulting in an overall symmetry of hemisphere function. All functional asymmetries would then be a result of anatomical asymmetries of the respective cortical regions (Berlucchi, 1983). In rebuttal Denenberg (1983) was forced to retreat to a valid but less interesting 'conceptual nervous system' position, where emphasis is on the nature of the resultant psychological functions rather than physiological mechanisms. He maintained that the net effect is mutual hemispheric inhibition, if the precise neuronal mechanism remains unknown.

As so often happens in debates on psychological topics, the physiologist – with his feet firmly planted on the ground – wins the argument but fails to address the most important questions! The physiological evidence for callosal inhibition is not as overwhelming as many psychologists would perhaps like to believe, but the behavioral evidence for *mutual inhibition* between the cerebral hemispheres, as marshalled by Denenberg, is strong enough that a simple excitatory model requires development precisely in the direction which the inhibitory models naturally lead. Without such development, the topographical excitatory model finds some support from cellular physiology, but appears to lack explanatory power in the realm of psychology. The most important issue which the excitatory model is incapable of directly dealing with is the fact that, together with massive increases in the size of the corpus callosum in *Homo sapiens*, there is a massive increase in the functional *asymmetry* of the brain. It may be possible to maintain that callosal size and cerebral asymmetry are totally unrelated issues, but the defenders of an excitatory callosal model must be able to explain how an excitatory tract has less and less of a tendency to produce bilateralization of function as it increases in size.

Denenberg's diffuse inhibitory hypothesis is the most formally developed model of this type. He assumes inherent functional asymmetries between the cerebral hemispheres of animals and man – asymmetries which can be augmented or reduced by early experience. The 'functional unit' of the brain in this view appears to be homologous cortical 'areas' connected by inhibitory callosal fibers such that normally one of the two areas is active and the other inactive. Denenberg does not pursue the neuronal physiology of this idea, but argues that various combinations of hemispheric activation (via brainstem routes) and callosal function can produce asymmetries in rats which are remarkably similar to those found in man. That is the left hemisphere is more easily activated in response to 'communicative functions,' whereas the right hemisphere 'will be selectively set to respond to spatial and affective information' (1981a, p. 15). With the 'activation' of either hemisphere, the contralateral hemisphere is inhibited callosally, thereby augmenting the functional differences between the left and right.

Denenberg's hypothesis has several attractions. It allows for the possibility of increased bilateralization of cortical functions – that is a suppression of callosal inhibition, which leads to the excitation of contralateral cortex. This he refers to as increased 'correlation' between the hemispheres. Moreover the level of hemispheric activation (fundamentally a subcortical effect) is a factor in determining the balance or dominance of the cerebral hemispheres. One minor criticism is that, while using words that can be construed to mean physiological processes, he is concerned primarily with the behavioral implications of 'activation,' 'inhibition' and 'correlation.' As discussed on pp. 91–111, I believe that some physiological detail can be added to the general framework of Denenberg's theory, but without that next level of detail the theory fails to draw the kind of explicit parallels between neuronal physiology and animal behavior which are needed for a mind/brain link of fundamental importance for psychology. It should also be noted that, being a 'diffuse' inhibitory model, it is unclear how information could be transferred across the corpus callosum.

On the other hand, Berlucchi's (1983) excitatory callosal hypothesis has all of the attractions of unambiguous cell physiology and must be considered the most likely explanation of callosal functions between regions of sensory cortex. Nevertheless without considerable amplification, the topographical excitatory hypothesis appears to explain little of the behavioral psychology which is at the heart of the laterality literature. Since he argues that the corpus callosum is centrally involved in 'yoking' the cerebral hemispheres and forcing them to work in unison, hemispheric specializations must therefore be seen as unique functions which have developed asymmetrically as a consequence of the *lack* of callosal input from the other side. In this view the callosum plays no active role in producing cerebral asymmetry.

The simplicity of this excitatory view of the corpus callosum is certainly an attraction but, again, it leaves a paradox concerning the simultaneous increases in callosal size and in functional asymmetries in the human brain. It is probably fair to say that the excitatory hypotheses in general are not designed, in the first place, to explain the functional differences between the hemispheres, but are more simply the most conservative extrapolations of lower-level physiological findings. Since most identified synapses in the brain are excitatory and the entire process of information transfer from the sensory organs to the cortex is fundamentally excitatory (with inhibition playing a role in 'sharpening' the percepts through a contrast-enhancement process), the safest guess concerning any nerve tract is that it is excitatory.

Once predominantly excitatory functions of the corpus callosum have been assumed, however, hemispheric asymmetries of function can be explained only in terms of inherent anatomical (neurotransmitter, etc.) differences, which themselves then need to be explained. Like much of reductionist theory, the danger of an infinite regress is real, but the attraction remains that certain kinds of questions are then deemed unimportant or 'bad questions.' 'Hemisphere' asymmetries then become differences in information processing among differently constructed neuronal 'modules' located in the left and right hemispheres; behavioral differences are then explained in terms of cellular or molecular differences. Needless to say, reduction of the complexities of one level to the relative simplicities of another level is laudable when genuine simplifications are obtained, but intolerable if the same unanswered questions are merely relegated to a different level.

THE DIFFUSE EXCITATORY HYPOTHESIS
The third school of thought concerning the corpus callosum is best represented by Guiard (1980), who has argued that the (implicitly excitatory) corpus callosum allows the active cortical modules in one hemisphere to 'alert' homotopic modules in the other hemisphere. Rather than the corpus callosum being involved in the transfer of information between the hemispheres, Guiard defends the unorthodox view that the callosum may be involved solely in the process of selective attention. The transfer of discriminatory learning between the eyes or limb extremities in various animal experiments (one example is given in chapter 6) is therefore thought possible due to brainstem routes, while the 'commissural system is the necessary mediator for the co-ordinated mobilization of the neuronal circuits on both sides of the cortex' (Guiard, 1980).

In his literature review of the transfer, integration and competition experiments in animals, Guiard has convincingly shown that many experiments which had previously been interpreted as demonstrating 'information transfers,' can as easily be interpreted as the effects of callosal 'arousal' or its absence. If, for example, the corpus callosum and optic chiasma are cut prior to unilateral training of one hemisphere, it is unclear, when subsequently testing the untrained hemisphere, whether or not the untrained hemisphere failed to learn the task because the specific information had not been shunted across the corpus callosum *or* because the untrained hemisphere was not provided with a callosal alerting stimulus during the training. If the relevant portion of contralateral cortex had been in effect 'asleep' during the training, then it may well be that any information sent to it by whatever route would not be recorded there.

The diffuse excitatory hypothesis also appears to avoid one of the theoretical problems raised by the diffuse inhibitory hypothesis. Why does the homotopic cortical module located contralaterally require suppression more than dozens of other competing modules located ipsi- or contralaterally? The predominantly homotopic nature of callosal fiber termination indicates that each cortical module is most concerned with communicating with its contralateral homolog, but why should this be within the framework of an inhibitory model? The diffuse excitatory model, on the other hand, requires homotopic callosal connections since the callosum is involved predominantly in the duplication of information in the two hemispheres – a role which would make sense only if each 'engram' contains similar ipsilateral connections. Functional asymmetries would therefore be a consequence of the failure to duplicate information – presumably due to asymmetrical hemispheric anatomy.

Several lines of evidence, however, argue against this view of callosal functions. A predominantly 'alerting' role of the corpus callosum suggests that callosumotomy should lead to increased bilateral *asymmetry*, but this has not been found in either psychological or physiological studies (see chapter 6). Moreover, an arousal-like role would also suggest that callosal fibers should terminate in a configuration similar to that of the non-specific brainstem fibers – i.e. in the superficial layers of the cortex. Particularly in primates, this is not the case (Jacobson and Marcus, 1970): callosal fibers terminate in the layer from which they originate – predominantly layers III and IV (although superficial termination and therefore a possible arousal role is the case in rodents).

Guiard's proposed reversal of arousal and informational functions is nonetheless an interesting and unconventional possibility which emphasizes one aspect of callosal activity which should be kept in mind. That is even if there are also mechanisms for the callosal transfer of information (by excitatory or inhibitory processes), the fact that the callosal effects are disynaptic indicates that they may have separate 'arousal' effects, unrelated to any informational effects. In other words, in addition to well-known brainstem mechanisms for arousal, corticocortical tracts in general and the forebrain commissures in particular may force two connected portions of cortex to work in parallel.

THE TOPOGRAPHICAL INHIBITORY HYPOTHESIS
Particularly prior to the elucidation of various anatomical asymmetries over the past twenty years, it appeared that the inhibitory models had

decisive advantages in explaining functional asymmetries of the cerebral hemispheres, but neither the excitatory nor the inhibitory models present any obvious explanations for the development of *complementary* asymmetries. The excitatory models suggest that callosal functions make the hemispheres *more* similar rather than less similar, and all empirical asymmetries must be explained in terms of inherent (anatomical, etc.) asymmetries. The diffuse inhibitory model unyokes the cerebral hemispheres and 'frees' them for separate development, but it does not produce lateral specializations which are necessarily related to one another. So while there may be no agreement concerning the basic mode of action of the corpus callosum, the two predominant schools of thought seem to favor the idea of *separate* hemispheric specializations – the one due solely to anatomical asymmetries of the hemispheres and the other due to the functional separation of the hemispheres caused by inhibitory forebrain commissures.

In contrast, the topographical inhibitory model explicitly accounts for *complementary* specializations. Details of this model will be outlined in the section which follows, but suffice it to say here that topographical inhibition shares with the topographical excitatory model the capability to transfer information across the corpus callosum and, at the same time, it shares with the diffuse inhibitory model the capability to produce and/or accentuate functional asymmetries of the hemispheres.

While not discussing neuronal mechanisms, Kinsbourne (1982) has developed one such view which emphasizes the importance of callosal inhibition in producing hemispheric complementarity. He argues that the approximate bilateral anatomical symmetry of the cerebral hemispheres and the approximate bilateral symmetry of subcortical arousal effects

> provides neural distance, not between alternative mutually exclusive acts, but between complementary component processes that combine to program a unitary pattern of behavior. By remaining separate until they are sufficiently elaborated to be combined, programs that contribute complementary elements maintain their differentiation and specificity.

In Kinsbourne's (1982) view the callosal connections prevent bilateralization and the duplication of information (by means of inhibitory effects) and therefore allow for the development and amplification of subtle information-processing differences which are due initially to the inherent biological differences between the cerebral hemispheres. Simultaneously in line with Guiard's hypothesis (1980), he argues that the commissures have an arousal effect such that, whenever one module in either hemisphere is actively processing information, its contralateral homolog is also at work. As Zaidel (1983) has commented, the corpus callosum according to Kinsbourne is a dynamic 'psychological factor,' whereas the hemispheric laterality effects are static and largely unalterable biological factors.

What then are those differences in information processing which each hemisphere is biologically favored to do? Kinsbourne suggests the following:

> As [an] object is scrutinized, glance by glance, touch by touch, two processes proceed in parallel. Information is extracted, serially, feature by feature; and concurrently, the location of each feature is registered on a centrally represented spatial framework, relative to the feature locations already represented. . . . The extraction of item and relational information is complementary: The former is typically left hemispheric and the latter typically right hemispheric.

We will return to this conception of hemispheric differences in the section which follows, and try to show more precisely how the corpus callosum plays an important role in its emergence.

Finally Doty and colleagues have advocated a somewhat different version of topographical inhibition as the likely mechanism of callosal function, based upon the results of animal experiments (Doty and Negrao, 1973; Doty et al., 1973; Doty and Overman, 1977; Doty et al., 1979). They have found that the anterior commissure and the corpus callosum exhibit different mechanisms for transferring information between the hemispheres of monkey brains. Whereas the anterior commissure allows for the excitatory transfer of information from one side to the other (bilateral engram formation), the corpus callosum allows only for 'access' to the information in one hemisphere by the other hemisphere – but not bilateral memories (unilateral engram formation). Since an intact corpus callosum allows for the transfer of specific information contained in one hemisphere, it could not be operating by means of diffuse inhibition or excitation, and since it does not allow for engram duplication, it could not be operating by means of topographical excitation. Since information does nonetheless pass over this nerve tract, the most parsimonious explanation of such results is that the corpus callosum is operating by means of topographical inhibition. We will return to this controversial topic in chapter 6.

The debate concerning the high-level functions of the corpus callosum seems to have come about this far (see chapter 6 also for a discussion of the role of the corpus callosum in stereoptic vision). On the one hand, the diffuse inhibitory model is more popular among psychologists, yet the topographical excitatory model has been favored by most physiologists. It is of interest, however, to note that neither of these relatively popular models requires consideration of subcortical mechanisms to understand the proposed callosal role of information transfer. In Denenbrg's model subcortical 'hemispheric activation' is an integral part of his theory, but activation is seen to function independently of information-transfer effects across the corpus callosum. On the other hand, Guiard's callosal activation model in a sense replaces subcortical arousal effects, such that the 'alerting' effect of the brainstem and the corpus callosum are similar.

In summary, most previous callosal hypotheses are concerned only with cortical functions unrelated to the rest of the brain. It might be argued that this simplicity in both theories is a commendable trait, but it might as easily be argued that both classes of model ignore very real subcortical effects which any realistic hypothesis of brain function must not omit. If indeed subcortical mechanisms of attention are at work and essential for conscious awareness of sensory stimuli reaching the cortex, then it may be dangerous oversimplification rather than laudable parsimony to exclude such processes in our first-order approximations. Again we are not in a position to decide this question on the basis of theoretical arguments, but comparison of these two hypotheses with the topographical inhibitory hypothesis, which demands consideration of subcortical attentional mechanisms highlights the possible significance of brainstem arousal processes even for the communication between the left and right cerebral cortices.

Further development of the topographical inhibitory hypothesis

By means of appropriate juggling of the starting premises of the above models of callosal function, the fundamental strengths of the topographical excitatory model and the diffuse inhibitory model can be incorporated within a hybrid theory, which I have called the topographical inhibitory model.

What is meant by 'topographical inhibition' (or equivalently 'homotopic inhibition') is inhibition via the corpus callosum of homotopic (mirror-image) cortical columns which are contralateral to active columns in the other hemisphere. The inhibition is likely to be disynaptic and to result in the inhibition of a cortical column (100–2,000 cells) which is the anatomical homolog of the activated column. 'Homotopic callosal inhibition' differs from 'diffuse callosal inhibition' precisely with regard to the area of contralateral cortex which receives the inhibitory effects. In most versions of the diffuse model, callosal inhibition is thought to have effects over large numbers of cortical columns – large enough to 'inactivate' or 'suppress' an entire region specialized for certain tasks. In the topographical inhibitory model, on the other hand, the inhibition is presumed to be effective only over the diameter of a single cortical column (<500 μm) – not over several millimeters or centimeters of contralateral cortex. Although the two models are in agreement with regard to the primary physiological effects of the corpus callosum, the homotopic inhibitory model alone appears to be consistent with the known fine-grained anatomy of callosal termination (which is also an essential part of the excitatory callosal model of Berlucchi).

Clearly most of the premises of a column-to-column inhibitory model are borrowed from either the topographical excitatory model or the diffuse inhibitory model. Specifically they include (i) approximate bilateral symmetry of the cerebral hemispheres (with small asymmetries favoring one hemisphere for language tasks); (ii) columnar organization of the neocortex; (iii) predominantly homotopic callosal connections (at least two per column); and (iv) monosynaptic or, more likely, disynaptic callosal inhibition of columnar activity. Finally both the excitatory and the inhibitory models presume (v) a unilateral superiority for speech production and comprehension, usually of the left hemisphere, due presumably to the need for unambiguous motor control over the organs of speech located on the midline of the body.

Two further assumptions are required in the topographical inhibitory model in order that it can account for the specifically *complementary* functions of the cerebral hemispheres: (vi) ipsilateral cortical surround inhibition among the cortical columns (an assumption which is implicit to most theories of cortical functioning). Finally, and most importantly since it is not a part of any of the other models, (vii) the topographical inhibitory model assumes a bilaterally symmetrical subcortical mechanism for arousal and attention.

Each of these premises requires further examination.

APPROXIMATE BILATERAL SYMMETRY OF THE CEREBRAL HEMISPHERES

Until the middle of the nineteenth century, the gross bilateral symmetry of the brain led to the assumption that the left and right cerebral hemispheres are functionally symmetrical and that their seemingly irregular and unquantifiable structural asymmetries are merely the normal statistical fluctuations reflecting individual differences, but not species-specific asymmetries. Not until the clinical demonstration of functional asymmetries in language production (1868) was there a forceful call to reconsider the 'complete symmetry' conception.

During the early twentieth century several studies demonstrated fairly stable anatomical asymmetries of the human brain, but not until a study by Geschwind and Levitsky in 1968 was an anatomical asymmetry of unquestionable significance reported. They found a portion of the left temporal lobe involved in auditory processing to be larger on the left in 65 percent, on the right in 11 percent and equal in 24 percent of their sample of 100 normal adults. These figures did not reach the 93 percent asymmetry that might have been expected from language dominance studies, but demonstration of an asymmetry near to Wernicke's area started the pendulum swinging in the other direction – some now believing that both hemispheres are collections of specialized 'modules' whose approximate anatomical symmetry is due to nothing more than the structural influences of the skull.

Empirically the cerebral asymmetries in man are now known to include the following (see Galaburda, 1984, for a more detailed review):

(i) *Superior temporal plane*: the surface area of the superior temporal plane (a portion of the superior temporal gyrus lying along the lateral fissure) is larger on the left than on the right in two-thirds of adult brains, with smaller percentages showing approximate symmetry or reversed asymmetry (Geschwind and Levitsky, 1968; Rubens, 1977; Galabruda et al., 1979). Moreover, this asymmetry is found in fetal brains as well (Wada et al., 1975). The largest asymmetry is at the posterior superior temporal gyrus (area 22).

(ii) *Parietal operculum*: LeMay and Culebras (1972) have reported a large left hemisphere parietal operculum (an extension of the post-central gyrus), which is the portion of somatosensory cortex which is involved in somesthetic perception of the articulatory apparatus.

(iii) *Frontal operculum*: the so-called frontal operculum, which is adjacent to or perhaps a part of Broca's area on the left, has been reported to be larger on the left than the right (Galaburda, 1984). Considered together, asymmetries (i), (ii) and (iii) suggest that the three cortical regions most intimately involved in the processing of linguistic material (the secondary auditory cortex, frontal cortex concerned with the motor control of the speech organs, and sensory perception of the changes in those organs) have larger representations in the left hemisphere.

(iv) *Hemisphere weight*: the right hemisphere is slightly heavier than the left (LeMay, 1976), possibly a consequence of the greater volume of white matter found on the right (Gur et al., 1983).

(v) *Frontal lobes*: the right frontal lobe is somewhat wider than the left (LeMay, 1976; Galaburda et al., 1979). Contrary to expectations, the pre-frontal cortex lying anterior of Broca's area (the so-called pars triangularis) is larger on the right than on the left, but this is conceivably a result of increased cortical space demanded by Broca's area itself.

(vi) *Occipital lobes*: the left occipital lobe is larger than the right one (LeMay, 1976) – again contrary to predictions if one assumes the right hemisphere to be dominant for visuospatial analysis.

(vii) *Thalamic neurotransmitters*: asymmetries of norepinephrine (Oke et al., 1978) and serotonin (Mandell and Knapp, 1979) have been demonstrated in several brainstem nuclei.

(viii) *Corticopyramidal tract*: a major subcortical asymmetry is found between the pyramidal tracts of the left and right which carry cortical information to the somatic musculature (Yakovlev and Rakic, 1966; Flor-Henry, 1983). That is more fibers descend from the left hemisphere to the right side of the body than vice versa and there is a relatively greater number of ipsilateral fibers traveling from the right hemisphere to the right musculature than vice versa. The fact that both hemispheres seem to conspire to produce greater control over the right-sided musculature suggests a fundamental, inherent anatomical origin for both left-sided control of speech and right-handedness.

As real as the above asymmetries are, and as important as they are for this or any theory of lateralization of functions (since left-sided language dominance and handedness are unambiguous empirical facts requiring an explanation), it must be noted that the bilateral asymmetries are nonetheless small when compared with differences between gyri, lobules or lobes in an anterior–posterior direction. The fundamental anatomical routes over which sensory information is supplied and retrieved are extremely similar on the left and right and, to varying degrees, quite different among different regions within a hemisphere. While the known asymmetries of the human brain may be only the tip of an iceberg of neuroanatomical asymmetries, it is nonetheless unlikely that the intrinsic or extrinsic connectivity of homologous cortical regions are fundamentally different. In other words, bilateral *symmetry* is the basic design of all brains from the tapeworm on up – with some small, albeit important, asymmetric variations added on. While some *quantitative* differences between the hemispheres are now known, fundamental *qualitative* differences would demand a degree of asymmetrical intrahemispheric connectivity which is simply unknown. It may not be possible to prove the negative argument, but the known symmetry of very simple invertebrate nervous systems and the conservative nature of evolution argue for asymmetries being *quantitative* differences in the numbers of cells or nerve fibers rather than *qualitative* rewirings (Braitenberg, 1977).

In conclusion left–right asymmetries undoubtedly play an important role in the emergence of slight superiorities on one side or the other, but the inherent differences in information processing between homologous cortical regions are nonetheless likely to be extremely small. While small asymmetries between homologous regions may produce an initial advantage in one hemisphere, alone a small quantitative difference between the cerebral hemispheres would not seem to be able to account for major qualitative differences between hemispheric capabilities.

We cannot afford to ignore the anatomical bilateral asymmetries of the brain any more than we can afford to overlook the biological 'asymmetries' between men and women, which historically have had such a pervasive effect on the social roles of the sexes. Nevertheless, for many purposes, it is precisely the extreme similarity between the left and right hemispheres (or between men and women) which will be of central importance when attempting to understand how they communicate. For biological reasons, the motivations of the left and right hemispheres may differ slightly, but they speak the same languages and, accepting some slight differences in talents and interests, are far more similar than dissimilar! As with differences between the sexes, we should neither dogmatically reject empirical findings of asymmetries (or 'inequalities') nor be so influenced by differences which barely creep into statistical significance that we conclude that they are two very dissimilar entities. For some reason, one hemisphere – usually the left – becomes the dominant 'executive' hemisphere when dealing with the external world, but the approximate bilateral symmetry – including virtually all tracts and nuclei – suggests that the two hemispheres process sensory information in similar ways.

Columnar organization of the neocortex

Do cortical columns really exist? The answer seems to be a qualified yes, but before reviewing the empirical evidence, let us consider the conceptual issues. In general it can be said that most psychologists accept the reality of cortical columns or some kind of cortical modularity as a logical necessity. To devise a theory of brain function based solely on four, six or even two hundred fundamental kinds of neurons – pyramidal cells, basket cells, interneurons, etc. – tends to place an unrealistically large demand on the information-processing capabilities of individual cells – the actual workings of which are fairly well understood and are not terribly psychological!

The analogous situation in computer science would be to discuss computer programs or artificial intelligence in terms of the resistors, transistors and other electronic components which are – from one point of view – all that computers really are. Particularly in computer science, all higher-level functions are made possible only by virtue of the engineer's complete understanding of the lower-level electronics, but it would be a futile, if not totally impossible task to discuss high-level functions in terms of the rock-bottom-level physics. Some higher-level structures (at least one level of code midway between the physics and the information-processing which allows for the representation of fundamental types of logical operations) is required as a functional unit to bridge the gap.

Perhaps more relevant than the computer analogy, however, is one from another of the natural sciences, cellular biology. The situation analogous to building a theory of brain functions from neuron units would be to try to develop a theory of cellular functions in terms of the atomic elements found in the typical cell. Certainly there is a small enough variety of atoms (around thirty) in the living cell to make possible a certain kind of characterization of cells in terms of atomic physics, but – with the exception of the ions which flow across semipermeable membranes – isolated atoms are only rarely encountered in the cellular milieu and are of importance only within the context of their interactions with large and complex molecules. So, when considering the fundamental processes of cellular life, our attention is inevitably drawn to the functions of the macromolecules, especially those of the nucleic acids and proteins, each of which contains hundreds or thousands of atoms.

As in cell biology, an understanding of the behavioral complexities of the animal organism depends crucially upon a basic understanding of the bits and pieces of the living organism – particularly the fundamental physiology of the neuron. A firm grasp of neuron science – the cellular 'atoms' of the brain is therefore the requisite starting-point, but it is unlikely that we will be able to draw many fruitful connections between the most fundamental physiological level (axons, pyramidal cells, dopamine, etc.) and high-level psychological events. Only once we have assembled the various physiological 'atoms' into some more capable functional units (whether cortical columns or some other analog of the cell's macromolecules) is it likely that parallels between physiological events and psychological events can be drawn.

For these reasons, the neurosciences require 'cortical column'-like, multi-neuron structures as the computing units of the brain. Just as the cell has come to be understood neither in terms of an unanalyzable 'life-force' nor in terms of the smallest atoms which comprise it, but rather in terms of (macro-) molecular biology, so the brain seems to require analysis neither as an impregnable, irreducible, mysterious 'black box' nor as a collection of cells, but rather as a system of relatively complex 'cell assemblies.'

Fortunately brain science has produced a likely candidate as the unit of brain functions in the discovery of the cortical column (figure 2.20). As noted in chapter 2, the usage of the phrase 'cortical column' varies and the smallest anatomical structure which is only 30 μm in diameter in visual cortex is not the same as the functional unit found elsewhere. Nevertheless the evidence for the functional and structural reality of such units (of varying sizes) is overwhelming (Mountcastle, 1978) and it would seem only a matter of time before precise definitions are available concerning the relationships between functional and structural units. For the skeptic, Mountcastle's (1978) review is an excellent place to start, although the criticisms of Towe (1975) are worth reading.

Figure 3.1 Anatomical indications of the columnar termination of callosal fibers interconnecting regions of premotor cortex in the monkey brain. (A) Injection of radioactively labeled amino acids to the right hemisphere resulted in the 'ocular dominance stripe'-like aggregation of the radioactivity in the homotopic cortex of the left hemisphere. These stripes are similar in terms of shape and size to those found in visual cortex. The dashed line indicates the rim of the so-called principal sulcus (from Goldman-Rakic, 1984). (B) Columnar structure evident in a cross-section through the principal sulcus (PS) at premotor cortex of the monkey brain. Two different kinds of label were used: horseradish peroxidase (HRP) was injected to the ipsilateral inferior parietal sulcus (IPS) and radioactive amino acids (H^3-AA) to the contralateral principal sulcus. Callosal fiber columns (2, 4, 5, 8, 10 and 11) and ipsilateral association fiber columns (1, 3, 6, 7 and 9) are seen to occupy separate regions of premotor cortex. It is noteworthy that columnar structure is evident throughout the six layers of the cortex.

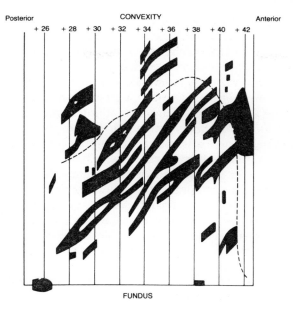

A

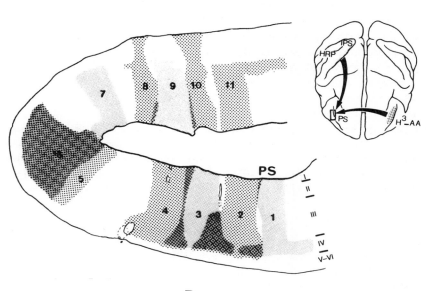

B

The congruence of three lines of evidence concerning columnar organization makes the case for a very widespread, general columnar organization of the cortex overwhelming. (i) Physiological evidence for columnar organization has been found in visual, auditory, somatosensory and motor cortex. Anatomical 'columns' have also been identified, but may not be identical with the physiological units. (ii) Columnar organization of a similar anatomical structure is seen in the termination of *callosal* fibers connecting regions of 'association' cortex (figure 3.1). (iii) Less explicit but of theoretical interest is the fact that the monoamine fibers from various lower brainstem nuclei terminate diffusely over most of the neocortex at intervals of about 100 μm. Whether or not the termination of the lower brainstem fibers is properly labeled 'columnar' is not certain, but the 100 μm spacing is of the appropriate dimensions to provide each cortical column with direct 'arousal' input from the brainstem. Together these three findings suggest the reality of columnar organization in sensory, motor and most importantly association cortex.

HOMOTOPIC CALLOSAL CONNECTIONS
Both gross anatomy and degeneration studies have shown an abundance of roughly homotopic connections between the cerebral hemispheres. Numerical estimates of the relative numbers of homotopic and heterotopic fibers have not been published, but the patterns of degeneration clearly indicate that more than three-quarters of callosal fibers are homotopic, while a large percentage of the heterotopic fibers go to limbic cortex. The significance of those limbic callosal fibers is not known, but it is of interest that, in cases of agenesis of the corpus callosum – instead of extending to the contralateral hemisphere – the callosal fibers form a bundle which runs within the ipsilateral cingulate gyrus and terminates in the ipsilateral olfactory system (Stefanko and Schenk, 1979) (see figure 4.3).

Figure 3.2 illustrates the homotopicity of callosal connections in the monkey brain, as demonstrated in a study by Hedreen and Yin (1981). The study involved injection of a small volume of an enzyme called horseradish peroxidase to the left inferior parietal cortex. Since the enzyme is known to be transported along neuronal axons to their sites of termination, the brain was excised after two days of survival and the location of the enzyme then studied. Following appropriate staining of the tissue, the contralateral cortex was seen to contain the enzyme in certain – predominantly homotopic – sites in the right inferior parietal cortex (figure 3.2(B)). Also illustrated in the figure are the layers of axonal termination – seen predominantly in layers III–V.

In a study focusing specifically on the question of the layering of callosal fibers, Jacobson and Marcus (1970) found that the pattern of termination differed among various species. In the monkey callosal fibers terminated primarily in layers IV and V, whereas in the cat there

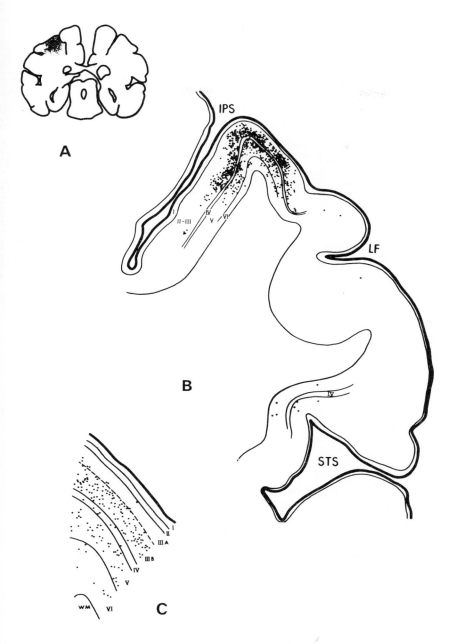

Figure 3.2 Homotopic callosal connections in the monkey brain. HRP injection to the left hemisphere (A) results in transport of the enzyme principally to the homotopic site in the right hemisphere (B). Some heterotopic fibers in the superior temporal sulcus (STS) and elsewhere in other cross-sections are evident, but the vast majority of callosal fibers are clearly homotopic. The origin and termination of most callosal fibers in the monkey brain are in layers IIIB through V (from Hedreen and Yin, 1981).

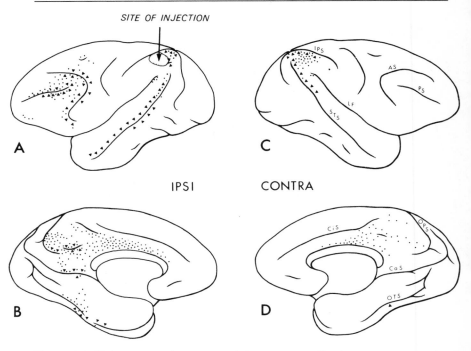

Figure 3.3 Homotopic and symmetrical heterotopic callosal connections in the monkey brain. Following HRP injection to the left hemisphere (A), the majority of callosal fibers are found to terminate at the homologous cortical region in the right hemisphere (C). Some of the ipsilateral association fibers in the left premotor cortex (A) do not have symmetrical callosal fibers (C), but some in the parietal and cingulate cortex (B) show symmetrical heterotopic callosal connections (D) (modified from Hedreen and Yin, 1981).

was a predominance in layers IIIA, IV and V, and in the rat primarily in the superficial layers, I and II. Most callosal fibers in all species originate in layer IV, but the species differences in termination undoubtedly signify species differences in function. At least in primates the predominance of termination in layers IV and V indicates that the homotopicity of callosal connections is not only to homologous cortical regions, but also to identical cortical layers. Termination in layers I and II may indicate a general 'arousal' function of the corpus callosum in lower species, since most of the nerve fibers from the lower brainstem nuclei terminate in those superficial levels.

Another unusual feature of callosal connections is not easily labeled as heterotopic or homotopic. That is in the case where strictly speaking heterotopic fibers are sent to the contralateral hemisphere, axonal transport is found ipsilaterally at a homotopic region. This pattern of connections, called symmetrical heterotopic connectivity, is illustrated in figures 3.3 and 3.4. The significance of symmetrical heterotopic

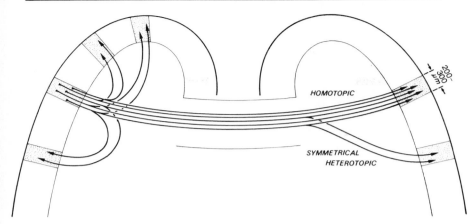

Figure 3.4 Schematization of 'homotopic' and 'symmetrical heterotopic' callosal connections. A cortical column will generally have more ipsilateral than contralateral connections and virtually all of its contralateral connections will find mirror-images in ipsilateral cortex.

connections is also not known, but they illustrate two important points concerning corticocortical communications: (i) there are precise and non-random connections between the hemispheres; (ii) assuming similar physiological effects of the 'symmetrical heterotopic' fibers and the ipsilateral association fibers, their inhibitory *or* excitatory activity would *increase* the similarity of activity of the two hemispheres. The same is not necessarily the case for strictly homotopic fibers: mutual inhibition would produce dissimilar hemispheric activity.

CALLOSAL INHIBITION

Stimulation of the corpus callosum itself or of regions of the neocortex has demonstrated a pattern of brief excitation at the site of termination of callosal fibers, followed by prolonged inhibition (figure 3.5). Since both physiological excitation and inhibition are known to occur, both the excitatory and the inhibitory hypotheses must be considered theoretical possibilities. Nevertheless the predominant effect appears to be inhibitory. Hossman (1975) notes: 'Of particular interest is the inhibitory phase following the transcallosal potential. . . . [The] delayed phenomena following transcallosal [excitation] should be the target of future research.' Some relevant animal studies on the physiology of the corpus callosum will be reviewed in chapter 6.

UNILATERAL SUPERIORITY OF ONE HEMISPHERE FOR SPEECH

The unilateral superiority of one hemisphere, usually the left, is one of the firmest empirical facts to be found in neuropsychology. Originally discovered from the loss of speech capabilities in patients with left-sided brain damage, the functional asymmetry of speech has now been

101

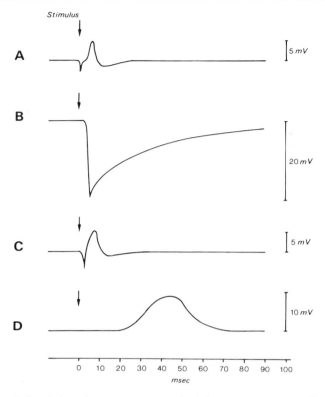

Figure 3.5 Callosal physiology. Excitatory and inhibitory responses to callosal stimulation are depicted in A and B respectively. The excitatory post-synaptic potential (EPSP) shown in A is rapid (monosynaptic), recovers rapidly and is only about 5 millivolts in amplitude. The inhibitory post-synaptic potential (IPSP) shown in B is slower to appear (disynaptic), recovers slowly over a period of 200 milliseconds and is about 20 millivolts in amplitude (after Toyama *et al.*, 1969). It is of interest to compare these two cortical responses with the excitatory events in the thalamus. In C, the response of cells in the specific 'relay' nuclei of the thalamus is seen to be rapid and excitatory, whereas those in the 'diffuse' reticular thalamic complex are more strongly excitatory, slower to begin and longer lasting.

demonstrated convincingly in three areas: (i) a large population of brain-damaged patients has been studied and the speech dominance of the left hemisphere in 93 percent of right-handers and 70 percent of left-handers has been confirmed; (ii) the Wada test (unilateral brain anesthetization) has been performed in a large sample of (non-trauma) neurological patients, again confirming the dominance of the left hemisphere in some 90 percent of right-handed subjects; (iii) unilateral presentation of stimuli to patients with severed forebrain commissures has shown that, in most cases, the left hemisphere is capable of responding verbally to stimuli received by it, whereas the right hemisphere is not. Moreover, based upon the techniques used in the split-brain studies, similar tests have been made of normal subjects – usually testing language comprehension rather than production – and again a left hemisphere superiority has been found. In summary, most people (particularly non-psychotic, right-handed males without familial sinistrality!) produce speech through the left hemisphere.

CORTICAL SURROUND INHIBITION

Cortical surround inhibition is known to occur in visual and somesthetic cortex. On theoretical grounds it is thought likely to occur elsewhere in the cortex (Walley and Weiden, 1973; Shallice, 1974) – probably anywhere that cortical columns are found, but its formal demonstration in motor, premotor and association cortex has not yet been possible. Empirically this is the weakest of the seven premises required for the topographical inhibitory model, but it is an implicit part of many discussions of cortical information processing and certainly has strong empirical support in primary sensory cortex. Lateral inhibition has been extensively documented at various cortical and subcortical stages in the sensory systems, particularly in vision. It is usually considered as a mechanism involved in enhancing contrast – that is making stimuli stand out against an inevitably noisy background. At least in visual cortex, an excitatory signal is normally surrounded by a region of inhibition (Hess et al., 1975) – with a maximum at 100–200 μm from the point of excitation. Although the precise mechanisms of such inhibition in the cortex are not certain, they may be due to short-range neural connections or dendrodendritic synapses (Shephard, 1974). Moreover it is worth mentioning that inhibitory callosal mechanisms have been suggested as a possible interhemispheric contrast-enhancement mechanism (Bava et al., 1970).

It is well known that surround inhibition is a common feature at all levels of *sensory* processing. For example, in the thalamus (LGN) of the cat, three kinds of cells involved with color-coding have been found with different center–surround relations. Most cells (77 percent) are type I, having a receptive field such that the cells are activated by a specific center color, but inhibited by an opponent color in the surround region. About 7 percent of the LGN cells show no distinct center–surround relationship (type II), whereas type III cells (16 percent) show an inhibitory response to any color, but an excitatory surround (or vice versa). See figure 3.6. Similar center–surround phenomena have been found at the cortical level, but generalization of this phenomenon to the entire (polymodal or supramodal) cortex remains problematical. Suffice it to say, that for the purposes of a topographical model of callosal functions, the demonstration of surround inhibition at other levels in the central nervous system suggests that a topographical model of callosal function may be viable.

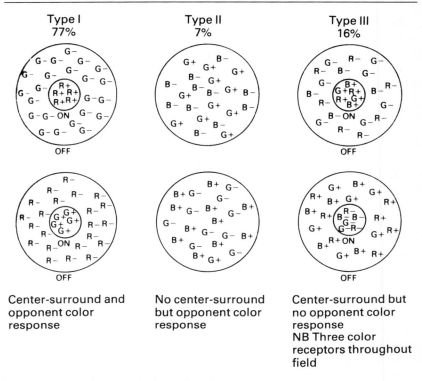

Figure 3.6 Center–surround relationships for color in the lateral geniculate nucleus of the cat brain (after Wiesel and Hubel, 1966). Type II cells do not show surround inhibition, but constitute a small percentage of cells, whereas other cells show color-specific surround inhibition (type I) or color non-specific surround inhibition or center inhibition–surround excitation (type III).

BILATERALLY SYMMETRICAL SUBCORTICAL MECHANISM OF AROUSAL

With regard to the question of the bilateral symmetry of subcortical arousal effects, it must first be acknowledged that some of the most interesting studies and virtually all of the publicity concerning hemisphere function have emphasized the *asymmetry* of the normally working brain. Not only as a consequence of several 'low technology' EEG studies, but also in the light of high technology brain imaging techniques (notably the PET scan), considerable attention has been drawn to the left–right *asymmetries* found in normal people when performing verbal or spatial tasks. Statistically significant differences in the activity of the two hemispheres have been reported in studies using the electroencephalograph (EEG, for example, Galin and Ellis, 1975), the so-called galvanic skin response (GSR, which measures essentially the amount of sweating on the hands; see, for example, LaCroix and Comper, 1979), and non-invasive techniques for measuring regional cerebral blood flow (rCBF; see, for example, Maximilian, 1982) and glucose metabolism (see, for example, Mazziotta *et al.*, 1982).

The importance of these studies for demonstrating the activation of relevant cortical subregions and functional asymmetries in normal subjects cannot be overstated, but these functional asymmetries should be considered within their proper contexts. In all cases the statistically significant bilateral asymmetries are small when compared against the magnitude of phasic changes or against the large differences which are found between anterior and posterior sites. Regardless of the psychologist's success or failure at inducing asymmetrical cognitive processing, there is an overall gross *symmetry* which must not be ignored.

While our interest may often lie with the positive (asymmetrical) results, it remains the case that in most of the reported EEG, rCBF and glucose consumption studies *where stimuli are presented bilaterally and unilateral motor activity is not allowed*, the left–right asymmetries are either extremely small or absent (e.g. Larsen *et al.*, 1978; Gevins *et al.*, 1979; Prohovnik *et al.*, 1980; Knopman *et al.*, 1982; and EEG studies reviewed by Donchin *et al.*, 1977). As real as some of the reported left–right differences undoubtedly are, in all cases the functional asymmetries constitute no more than a few percent disparity between remarkably similar measures of cortical activity (see, for example, figures 3.7 and 3.8). In other words, virtually all physiological measures which might be construed as reflecting the quantitative level of arousal of the cerebral hemispheres show fairly constant bilateral symmetry, while at the same time absolute levels and anterior/posterior ratios vary considerably.

Similar conclusions can be drawn from the anatomy and physiology of subcortical structures. On the one hand, the asymmetric functioning of the so-called *specific* nuclei of the thalamus, as determined by direct stimulation (Ojemann, 1977), indicates an asymmetry of function which correlates well with the known functional asymmetries of the neocortex. That is stimulation on the left is far more disruptive of language production or comprehension than is stimulation on the right. The non-specific or diffuse thalamic nuclei, on the other hand, constitute the rostral end of the reticular activating system, which has extensive bilateral connections throughout the brainstem. Although the degree of bilateral cortical projections from the diffuse thalamic nuclei decreases with phylogenetic ascendency (Scheibel and Scheibel, 1967), unilateral stimulation of any part of the reticular activating system will produce bilateral effects (French, 1973). Stimulation of lower brainstem monoamine nuclei also results in bilateral cortical activation, as would be predicted from the bilateral coursing of brainstem cholinergic fibers. Finally the so-called thalamic adhesion is present in some 70 percent of human brains and allows for interhemispheric communication between non-specific midline nuclei.

It can therefore be said that one of the strongest arguments against

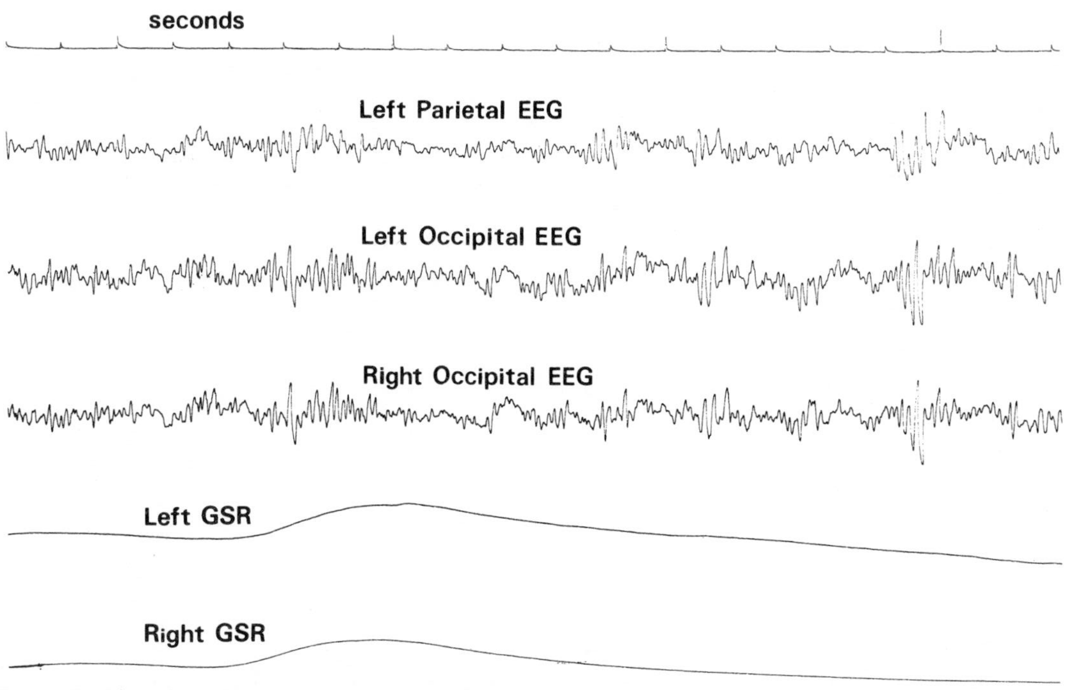

Figure 3.7 Physiological evidence of the bilateral symmetry of the cerebral hemispheres. A typical recording of the electroencephalograph (EEG) and galvanic skin response (GSR) in a normal subject at rest. The left occipital electrode was positioned equidistant between the left parietal and right occipital electrodes. It is evident from both the raw trace and spectral analysis that the electrical activity is more similar between homologous sites over the left and right hemispheres than between two similarly spaced sites within a single hemisphere. The GSR is a peripheral measure of brain activity which typically shows bilateral symmetry in the changes in sweating at the fingertips of the left and right hands – indicative of bilateral arousal of the autonomic nervous system.

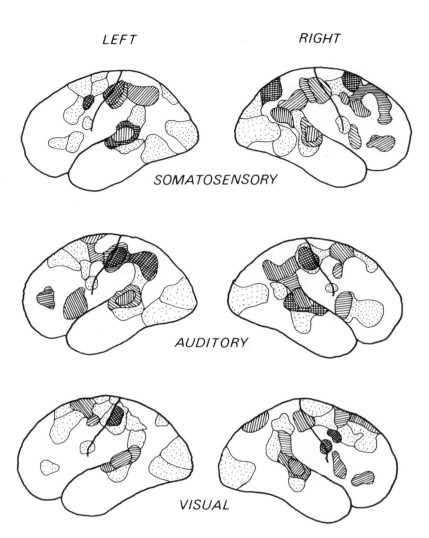

LEFT   RIGHT

SOMATOSENSORY

AUDITORY

VISUAL

Figure 3.8 Recordings of regional cerebral blood flow in normal subjects receiving somatosensory, auditory or visual stimulation (adapted from Mazziotta *et al.*, 1982). These findings were reported as showing differences in activation according to the sensory modality and as indicating hemispheric specializations depending upon the task. When stimuli were presented unilaterally, stronger left–right asymmetries were found (results not shown), but when a more natural *bilateral* presentation was used, laterality effects were small. The density of the cross-hatching and stipling indicates the percentage increase in cerebral blood flow relative to a rest condition.

the *diffuse* inhibitory model of the corpus callosum, i.e. the lack of physiological asymmetries comparable to the asymmetry of language functions (Berlucchi, 1983), constitutes support for the *topographical* inhibitory theory, which requires bilateral cortical arousal for the flow of information between the cerebral hemispheres.

The seven points summarized above serve not only to illustrate the fundamental strengths of the topographical inhibitory hypothesis, they also point out several trouble-spots for the alternative hypotheses.

As summarized in table 3.1 the topographical excitatory theory alone can explain little of the empirical findings on cerebral laterality. At the very least, the excitatory theory requires consistent anatomical asymmetries to explain asymmetrical functions of the cerebral hemispheres and, thus far, the evidence on both anatomical and neurotransmitter asymmetries provides some indication of small differences, but as yet no suggestion of drastically different modes of information-processing. Even with a much stronger correlation between behavioral asymmetries and anatomical asymmetries than is currently known, how anything beyond small quantitative differences between the hemispheres could emerge and what the role of the corpus callosum might be remain far from clear in such a view. If each hemisphere can be characterized as a collection of anatomically specialized 'modules,' why is commissural input of any importance at all in higher cognitive processes, and why should there be steadily increasing commissural input as we ascend the phylogenetic scale? Perhaps these questions can ultimately be answered within the framework of the excitatory hypothesis, but considerable theoretical elaboration on the mechanisms of excitatory callosal functions will be required.

All of the inhibitory hypotheses, on the other hand, appear to be consistent with the major thrust of the findings concerning lateral specialization and the effects of callosal dysfunction (table 3.2). With the further assumptions required for the topographic inhibitory hypothesis, the inhibitory view of the corpus callosum appears to be consistent with (i) the basic anatomical and physiological constraints of the cortex and (ii) the major behavioral findings of callosal transection and agenesis (chapter 4). Although explicit demonstration of *topographical* callosal inhibition at the cellular level has not been achieved, the behavioral evidence and physiological plausibility of the hypothesis suggest that a 'mirror-image negative,' as opposed to a 'carbon-copy' relationship between the cerebral hemispheres, is possible.

It is worth emphasizing that, insofar as cortical regions communicate via topographical mapping, logically a second area can receive *information* from a first area in only two ways: either as a 'carbon-copy' replication of a specific configuration of neuronal excitation, or as a 'photographic negative.' Carbon-copy transmission of topographical information is the established rule in relaying sensory information from the sense organs to at least secondary sensory cortical areas – and

Table 3.2 Theoretical issues related to callosal functions

	Homotopic excitatory theory	Diffuse inhibitory theory	Homotopic inhibitory theory
Anatomy	Major and consistent asymmetries predicted to produce behavioral asymmetries. Human anatomical asymmetries are not consistent enough or even indicate the correct direction in some cases. Animal asymmetries would suggest more behavioral asymmetries than now known.	Callosal termination is too narrow (about 300 μm) to allow for diffuse callosal inhibition. Other mechanisms required, but diffuse inhibition would imply large physiological asymmetries which have not been found.	Anatomical asymmetries not predicted and find no natural place in the theory. Anatomical asymmetry resulting in unilateral speech capacities is essential but other asymmetries remain unexplained (i.e. must be viewed as the statistical variation in normal brains without any fundamental significance).
Physiology	Prolonged inhibitory effect of callosal stimulation not accounted for.	The brief excitatory effect of callosal stimulation not accounted for.	The brief excitatory effect of callosal stimulation not accounted for.
Importance	'Unifies' the left and right sides of the brain by forcing them to act in unison.	'Frees' the right hemisphere to develop independent specializations, but what does 'freed' mean?	Essential for right hemisphere 'complementarity' to left hemisphere functions. Important mechanism of cognitive generalization; essential for normal intelligence.
Unilateral speech functions	Unilateral engram formation in response to bilateral sensory input in human language comprehension remains unexplained. Anatomical asymmetries required.	Unilateral engram formation requires some prior advantage of one hemisphere. Inhibitory callosum augments hemispheric asymmetry.	Unilateral engram formation requires some prior advantage of one hemisphere. Inhibitory callosum augments hemispheric asymmetry.

perhaps beyond, ipsilaterally. Further 'carbon-copy' transmission in primary visual and primary auditory cortex is also likely but, as will be discussed more fully in chapters 4 and 6, both clinical and experimental studies have indicated that (i) the corpus callosum transfers information between the cerebral cortices, but (ii) not of sufficient strength or appropriate nature to establish identical engrams bilaterally. The unilaterality of at least some kinds of information storage is most clearly demonstrated in the unilaterality of human speech capacities. Topographical callosal excitation cannot explain this phenomenon, and topographical callosal inhibition provides the first logical alternative mechanism of interhemispheric communication.

Although the idea of callosal *inhibition* has frequently been considered as essential to explain hemispheric specialization (e.g. Kinsbourne, 1974; Denenberg, 1981) and abnormalities of specialization (e.g. Flor-Henry, 1979a) and although *mirror-image* transfer via homotopic commissural fibers has been invoked to explain lateral mirror-image confusions in children and animals (e.g. Orton, 1937; Noble, 1968; Corballis and Beale, 1976), the possibility of a *mirror-image negative* relationship has not previously been explored. If, however, the cerebral hemispheres are predominantly symmetrical and connected homotopically, then the mirror-image negative is one of only two possible topographical relationships between them.

In summary the topographical inhibitory model of callosal function is based upon seven premises concerning the cerebral cortex, the non-specific 'arousal' mechanisms of the brainstem and the corpus callosum itself. Most of those premises appear to be well established. The corpus callosum connects primarily homotopic regions of the two hemispheres and its strongest physiological effect is inhibitory. The cerebral cortex has a columnar texture, such that callosal fibers are likely to influence the functioning of 'cortical cylinders' containing 100–1,000 cortical neurons. Such cylinders are known to have inhibitory effects on their nearest neighbors in sensory and motor regions of the cortex and, on theoretical grounds, are thought likely to have similar effects over association cortex. Subcortical arousal effects are generally, if only approximately, bilateral in nature. Consequently whenever bilaterally symmetrical patches of the cerebral cortex are activated by such brainstem mechanisms, a mirror-image negative relationship between the cerebral hemispheres would be produced by an inhibitory corpus callosum. If either hemisphere is 'dominant' for a function and produces, for example, a unilateral motor engram, then an inhibitory corpus callosum would produce a contralateral 'contextual' engram.

According to the topographical inhibitory model, therefore, the difference between the activity in the left and right hemispheres will be the difference between a focus of activity, on one side of the brain, and its immediate surround with the focus deleted, on the other side. In terms of human language, two essentially identical (homotopic) regions of cortex on the left and right will contain essentially identical linguistic information, but a topographical inhibitory relationship between them implies that the explicit, denotative language on one side will be suppressed contralaterally. Simultaneously the effects of reduced surround inhibition from the inhibited region will result in an increase of 'other' linguistic elements – which are, in a functional sense, closely related to the linguistic focus in the contralateral hemisphere. In this way the hemisphere which is 'non-dominant' for language will be actively processing linguistic material which has related cognitive content, although the precise pattern in the 'dominant' hemisphere will not be duplicated in the 'non-dominant' hemisphere. As such, the non-language hemisphere will be actively and continually involved in the processing of the connotations, implications and linguistic ramifications of the denotative language in the left.

In general the difference in the cognitive content of the two hemispheres will be between linguistic denotation and paralinguistic connotation – between explicit relationships among objects and events as specified through language, on the one hand, and classes of similar relationships, on the other hand. As an aside, it is worth mentioning that, insofar as parallel associational fibers connect various cortical regions, this mechanism of 'cognitive generalization' may not be unique to cortical regions joined by the corpus callosum; it could be an ongoing process wherever *inhibitory* fibers join two regions with cortex and where there are appropriate mechanisms for subcortical arousal.

Due solely to the extensive bilateral connections throughout the brainstem in general and the reticular activating system in particular, arousal effects are approximately bilateral in most normal situations. For this reason the 'focus/context' relationship between the cerebral hemispheres will be an ongoing, virtually continuous process of hemispheric complementarity. In contrast the simultaneous arousal of two *intra*hemispheric regions would be possible (given appropriate arousal mechanisms), but not as inevitable as the simultaneous arousal of homotopic sites on the left and right. It therefore seems likely that the mirror-image negative mechanism of corticocortical communication may be a common and inevitable aspect of *inter*hemispheric communications, whereas it may occur less frequently *intra*hemispherically.

In contrast to previous inhibitory models, the mirror-image negative relationship between the cerebral hemispheres implied by the topographical inhibitory model suggests that a unilateral engram would 'switch off' only its own precise mirror-image contralaterally. Column-by-column homotopic inhibition implies a complementary pattern which, although doubly transformed into a mirror-image negative and inevitably degenerate, nonetheless contains topographical neural information which is complementary to that in the other hemisphere. In other words, whichever hemisphere is *not* dominant for language (due presumably to anatomical or biochemical asymmetries) would contain complementary contextual information which, although not amenable to precise and coherent expression, entails cognitive processing at a level comparable to that of language itself.

Despite minor superiorities of one hemisphere or the other in terms of speed or precision, the bilateral symmetry of all sensory pathways and the continuous commissural 'yoking' of one hemisphere to the other will imply that sensory information stored at the cortical level will be virtually identical on both sides. Thus only in motor processes such as speech (where there is competition for midline organs) will there occur unilateral activation of cortical columns involved in the premotor preparation and actual motor act itself. Due to callosal inhibition, speech would activate contralateral cortical columns which do not constitute an identical engram, but rather an engram which is, at each instant of cortical processing, the spatial complement of the motor engram.

Computer simulation of callosal effects

The psychological implications of the three main hypotheses concerning the functions of the corpus callosum will be examined in chapter 4, but it is instructive to make a comparison of the expected effects on cortical activation predicted by each hypothesis. For this purpose, the results of two elementary computer simulations will be discussed (program details are in appendix 2). The first simulation deals solely with the nature of the spatial patterns of cortical activity which each callosal hypothesis implies and the second simulation concentrates on the temporal changes which are found in two 'neural nets' which contain both extensive intra- and inter-net connections. Neither simulation demonstrates what real brains can or cannot do, but they are useful exercises for demonstrating the logic of how complex patterns can arise from essentially simple neural interactions.

For the purposes of simulation one, the cortex is assumed to be comprised of cortical columnar units which are close-packed in a hexagonal array over the entire surface of the cortex (figure 3.9). The excitatory influences on any given column are assumed to arrive via corticocortical fibers and via subcortical 'arousal' fibers. The excitatory influences from sensory organs and other cortical areas are presumed to be 'informational' effects – causing the transmission of a pattern of activity in response to an informational event at another site, whereas the 'non-specific' brainstem excitatory influences are presumed to be more diffuse effects which increase the base level of activity in a given cortical region, but which are not in themselves 'informational.' This distinction between informational and non-informational cortical activity is somewhat artificial – particularly insofar as the results of the computer simulation must be evaluated either in terms of the two-dimensional pattern of activation or the temporal changes in activity –

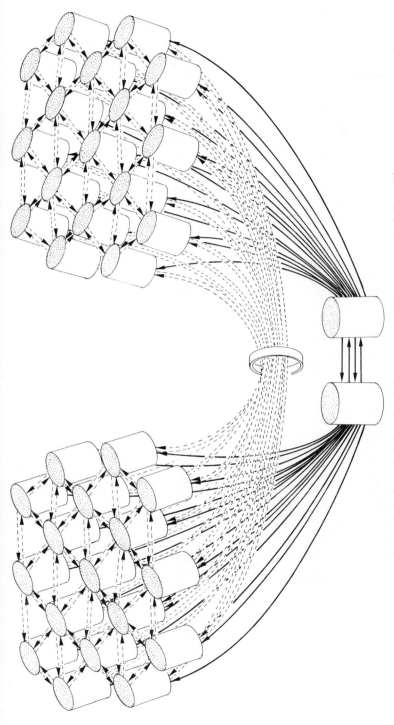

Figure 3.9 A portion of the cortical structure assumed for computer simulations. The cortical 'cylinders' are in a hexagonal close-packed array and are connected afferently and efferently with contralateral homologous cylinders. All cortical cylinders receive excitatory and inhibitory input.

unrelated to the 'information' which such activation may convey. It is nevertheless important conceptually to distinguish between specific and nonspecific thalamic input – the former carrying patterned sensory information about the external sensory field and the latter 'activating' portions of such cortical information.

It is further assumed that all cortical columns have inhibitory effects on their six nearest neighbors. The spatial and temporal dimensions of such inhibitory effects can be adjusted within the simulation, but are not central to the demonstration of complementary cortical patterns due to callosal effects.

Simulation one is based upon two patches of cortical columns, as illustrated in figure 3.9. Assuming that the functional unit of the brain is two cortical columns in the left and right cerebral hemispheres and their callosal connections, the patterns of activity generated by various kinds of callosal assumptions can be studied. Representative outputs are shown in figure 3.10.

Whereas simulation one is entirely static (spatial) in its representation of two patches of cortex, simulation two is temporally dynamic, but simplified in the spatial dimensions. That is an array of cortical neurons is generated which is made to change with time as a function of previous states. The interconnections among the cortical units are based upon specified percentages of excitatory and inhibitory inputs, but their two-dimensional spatial locations are not taken into account. The output of simulation two concerns the continuing summation of excitatory states and whether or not cyclic activity in the nets is generated. Representative results with various percentages of inhibitory and excitatory connections can be found in appendix 2.

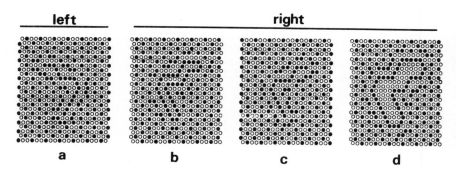

Figure 3.10 Typical cortical patterns produced in the simulation by three hypotheses concerning callosal function. On the left (a) is shown a pattern of cortical activity which is generated unilaterally in the left hemisphere – such as that produced, for example, in the generation of speech. On the right are shown the patterns of cortical activity in the right produced by (b) homotopic callosal excitation, (c) homotopic callosal inhibition, and (d) diffuse callosal inhibition. See appendix 2 for further details.

114

Homotopic callosal inhibition implies that the activity of a cortical column in one hemisphere will inhibit the activity of its contralateral homolog for a given period of time (the specified post-synaptic inhibitory potential). Surround inhibition will imply ipsilateral suppression of columnar activity for a comparable time period. Furthermore, given the decrease in firing contralaterally (i.e. contralateral surround inhibition) there will be less inhibition across the corpus callosum and therefore more ipsilateral firing. The degree of activity in 'surround columns' will be proportional to the degree of subcortical arousal effects and inversely proportional to the degree of callosal inhibition.

In summary simulation one demonstrates that a few extremely simple rules concerning cortical column interactions can generate mirror-image reversals and photographic-like negation. Simulation two shows that cyclic activity can be generated by a randomly connected net provided that there is not excessive excitation or inhibition entering the system. A more realistic attempt at simulating the cortex would require greater attention to the simultaneous spatial and temporal connectivity of the cortical units, but this topic will not be pursued here (see Anninos and Cook, 1986).

The significance of these computer exercises is that they demonstrate how two *identical* cortical 'nets' with *identical* dynamics within each net can nevertheless exhibit different patterns of activation due to the connectivity between them. Given an initial asymmetry of activation, such as is presumed to occur in speech, we are not therefore faced with a choice between roughly symmetrical hemispheric activation (the excitatory callosal hypothesis) or grossly asymmetric 'on-off' patterns of activation (the diffuse inhibitory callosal hypothesis). On the contrary, we are able to generate relatively small asymmetries due solely to callosal activity and we avoid all speculation about different hemispheric 'modes of information processing' which would imply fundamentally different neuronal mechanisms in the left and right.

It remains to be seen how important these asymmetries might be for cognition, but the differential activation of a bilaterally represented semantic net can be easily seen. If each node in the nets shown in figure 3.9 is given a unique lexical meaning and its strength of association with other nodes specified, then activation of a portion of the lexicon on one side will lead to complementary activation contralaterally (see figure 4.1). With repeated generation of speech from the left hemisphere, it is easy to see how a tonic denotation–connotation dichotomy could arise in the cerebral hemispheres.

The generation of higher-order dichotomies is more complex, but might occur in a similar fashion. That is, as the left hemisphere puts together lexical strings, the right hemisphere would receive more diffuse activation of words related to the left-sided phrases, thus activating more strongly the superordinate concepts involved. For example, if the left hemisphere were to generate 'the red shirt', callosal inhibition of 'red' would *disinhibit* its near neighbors in the semantic net ('orange', 'purple', 'green', 'blue', etc.) in the right hemisphere. If there were excitatory links between each color and the superordinate concept of 'color', then there would be more activation of the concept in the right hemisphere than in the left. A similar situation would exist with regard to 'shirt', where 'trousers', 'socks', 'sweater', etc, would be *inhibited* in the left and *excited* in the right. The superordinate concept of clothes would therefore be more strongly activated in the right hemisphere. In this way, the explicit verbal information would be far more strongly recorded in the left hemisphere, but the right hemisphere would in fact end up with a better idea of the underlying concept, 'colorful clothes'.

Summary

There are currently four principal models concerning the role of the corpus callosum. Each perspective has some theoretical advantages and some supporting physiological evidence and indeed each may be valid at different parts of the cortex or even in different animal species. A notable weakness of the topographical excitatory model is its reliance upon morphological asymmetries to explain all forms of lateral specialization and simultaneously its lack of a *raison d'être* for the corpus callosum. A notable weakness of the diffuse inhibitory model is the lack of physiologically demonstrable asymmetries of cortical arousal. A notable weakness of the excitatory arousal model is the lack of an explanation for hemisphere differences and the need to postulate inherent differences in hemispheric 'information-processing.' The topographical inhibitory model is thought to avoid these problems and to exhibit most of the strengths of the three previous models. Specifically these strengths can be summarized as follows:

(i) Hemispheric functional asymmetries are due at least partially to callosal effects – thus avoiding the need for a perfect correlation between anatomical and functional asymmetries.

(ii) The corpus callosum has a dual role – the unification of the bilateral sensory and motor fields and the generation of asymmetrical cortical information.

(iii) Only minimal metabolic and physiological asymmetries are expected (as frequent and consistent as anatomical asymmetries, but not approaching an 'on–off' asymmetry).

(iv) Differences in hemispheric information-processing are due to: small anatomical asymmetries and persistent hemispheric complementarity due to callosal inhibition.

As will be discussed in great detail in the chapter which follows, the 'focus/context' conception of hemispheric specializations has the principal merit of offering a physiologically precise mechanism by which *complementary* hemispheric functions might be produced. A similar psychological dichotomy for the cerebral hemispheres has been advocated by several of the leading psychologists investigating cerebral laterality, most notably Kinsbourne (1982), who has commented as follows:

> The right hemisphere fits successive acts of information extraction . . . into a framework that is based upon the initial overview of the scope of the problem and makes it possible, by preserving the unbalancing effect of the shifting focus of attention, by holding it in context. At the level of scholarship also, the holding in context of successive advances in understanding has obvious merit!

Could an inhibitory corpus callosum be the underlying mechanism which results in the cerebral hemispheres accomplishing such complementary functions?

4

NEUROPSYCHOLOGICAL IMPLICATIONS OF CALLOSAL FUNCTION

The three preceding chapters have reviewed the fundamental anatomical and physiological findings which must underlie any theory of callosal function and hemispheric specialization. First of all, we have found that the cortex of each cerebral hemisphere must be considered as a two-dimensional surface on to which many 'maps' of the external world are projected. Some of those maps are well understood and correspond in a sensible way with the two-dimensional configuration of sensory organs. Other maps appear to be distortions or partial representations of the 'primary' maps, and still other portions of sensory cortex do not appear to exhibit topographical maps.

Including a large portion of the frontal lobes, it must be said that the organizational pattern of much of the cortex remains unknown, but – at the very least – we have a good understanding of sensory topographical mapping, and can reasonably extrapolate some possibilities concerning polymodal maps. It seems likely that there also occurs some form of abstract 'supramodal' sensory mapping. The mechanisms of such supramodal mapping are unknown, but until given some contradictory findings, we might safely assume that the processing of abstract information will involve the same kinds of topographical transformations which are found in the projection and manipulation of the motor and sensory maps. In other words, whatever the nature of 'abstract' information-processing, it is likely to occur on a two-dimensional cortical surface and to be subject to most of the anatomical and physiological restrictions which operate in sensory cortex.

Secondly, tabulation of the numbers of cortical columns and commissural fibers suggests that, particularly in the more advanced mammals, there is a sufficient number of callosal fibers to connect large portions of the neocortex column-by-column between the left and right cerebral hemispheres. Precisely how homologs on the left and right might be affecting each other remains a controversial question, but the abundance of callosal fibers and their homotopic connectivity clearly suggest a few elementary kinds of topographical transformations of cortical information across the corpus callosum.

Based upon these anatomical considerations, three contrasting perspectives on callosal functions have been identified and their predictions

118

can now be compared against empirical findings on the neuropsychology of normal and abnormal brains.

Normal functions of the corpus callosum in the intact brain

Perhaps the *least* conclusive of all the arguments concerning callosal function are based upon findings on the normal, intact brain. This is a paradox pervading all of neuropsychology: it is far easier to determine what a brain cannot do once a portion of it has been damaged than it is to determine what that portion can do while still present. We are led into a kind of reversed logic in which the functions of a region or tract can be deduced only when they are gone. For this reason, patients in which the corpus callosum is severed or absent from birth, and patients with unilateral brain damage (see pp. 124–44) will probably provide the conditions most suitable for testing hypotheses concerned with callosal functions. Nevertheless the most interesting questions are concerned with the normal functions of the corpus callosum in the normal brain and at least tentative conclusions can be drawn from experiments in normal subjects and from some rather general considerations of the brain.

When the intact brain is to be studied, however, there are technical limitations on the stimulation and measurement of responses on one side of the brain or the other. Even when using direct physiological means for measuring brain activity, problems inevitably arise with regard to the limitations of spatial or temporal resolution. The electroencephalograph (EEG) and magnetoencephalograph (MEG) are electromagnetic measures and therefore can be recorded with as much temporal precision as desired (theoretically up to the speed of light), but the spatial resolution is poor and there is even debate concerning whether a visual evoked potential recorded over the occipital cortex of one hemisphere reflects the ipsilateral or the contralateral cortex more strongly! In contrast glucose metabolism and regional cerebral blood flow (rCBF) techniques provide impressive spatial resolution (less than 1 centimeter), but normally require summation over a period of several minutes – a time during which the subject might experience a variety of different and contradictory psychological states!

For these and other reasons, most research on normal subjects has been done using visual half-field (tachistoscope) and dichotic listening techniques. Here again there are technical problems. When a light stimulus is presented to a unilateral visual field, the eyes naturally realign on the stimulus within a few milliseconds, thus sending it to both hemispheres. Consequently only extremely brief periods of presentation can be used. Rapid presentation effectively produces unilateral stimulation, but simultaneously drastically limits the complexity of the stimuli which can be used. Clearly this limitation does not adversely affect studies designed to examine recognition speeds, thresholds of perception or reaction times, but if we are interested in the contribution of one hemisphere or the other to the understanding of, for example, metaphors, then the brevity of tachistoscopic presentation is a serious shortcoming. As valid as conclusions using such methods may be, they can tell us only about certain aspects of hemisphere functioning under certain unusual and quite unnatural conditions. Under normal circumstances the two hemispheres would hardly ever receive sensory information which is even mildly incongruent, much less contradictory. And although brains can be studied in terms of perceptual thresholds and reaction times, our conscious minds in normal situations are more often involved in deciphering metaphors than in detecting flashes of light!

On the other hand, presentation of normal (bilateral and slow) stimuli – as is the usual case in a natural setting – cannot allow us to draw any conclusions about hemisphere differences simply because the callosal transmission of nervous impulses from one hemisphere to the other occurs in less than 10 milliseconds. (And who knows how many times such communication would occur before we get around to our typically lethargic 500 millisecond motor responses?) For this reason, neuropsychological research on normal subjects has become subdivided into three areas: (i) psychophysiological techniques, principally the EEG, with its poor spatial resolution; (ii) 'scanning' and blood flow techniques, principally glucose metabolism and regional cerebral blood flow methods, with their poor temporal resolution; and (iii) split-field techniques, principally tachistoscopic and dichotic methods, with their unnatural stimulus presentation.

Among the split-field studies the vast majority has been concerned with the manipulation of rather simple stimulus characteristics in order to deduce a 'fundamental' dichotomy of hemispheric information-processing (see chapter 5), but some of the most interesting studies have been done on clearly high-level information processing. One such study was that of Regard and Landis (1984), who presented short words to the left or right visual fields for extremely brief periods (5–25 msec) and had their normal subjects read the words which they had just seen. With the presentation speed adjusted for each subject such that only one-quarter of each subject's answers was correct, some interesting findings were obtained concerning the nature of the mistakes which were made in relation to the side of presentation. In comparison with the left hemisphere, the right hemisphere had a highly significant tendency to make mistakes called 'semantic paralexias.' That is, the word was not read correctly, but a word with a related meaning was substituted. Although the two hemispheres were equally inaccurate in misreading words due to letter substitutions or in being unable to see any word at all, the substitution of an incorrect word with a related meaning was more often done by the right hemisphere.

This phenomenon of semantic paralexia in normal subjects is of interest because a similar condition is found among some patients with left hemisphere damage, a subgroup of the so-called deep dyslexics (Coltheart, 1983). Some such patients are found to have grossly impaired reading skills, but – interestingly – they show a tendency to misread words by substituting words with related meanings. It has thus been argued that this unusual reading capacity may be achieved by the right hemisphere. The topic of deep dyslexia remains controversial, but clearly such patients pose a problem for those who would assign virtually all higher-level cognitive skills to the left hemisphere. Not only can the right hemisphere contribute to the process of reading, but also it is capable of a high-level comprehension of the written word.

The demonstration by Regard and Landis of a similar phenomenon in normal subjects seems to indicate that semantic paralexia is *not* an anomaly produced by a grossly abnormal brain, but a *normal* semantic ability of the right hemisphere which can be uncovered only through brain damage or unusually rapid stimulus presentation. The Regard and Landis study is one of a very small number done on normal subjects to examine right hemisphere semantic capabilities. Most studies using the tachistoscope have in fact demonstrated vast superiorities of the left hemisphere in detecting and decoding phonemes and graphemes and in translating one system into the other. While the linguistic talents of the left hemisphere seem well established in light of such findings, those unilateral superiorities do not give us many clues concerning the validity of the various callosal hypotheses.

So how might the semantic paralexias shed light on callosal functions? The fact that the right hemisphere has some impressive semantic capabilities does not find an easy explanation in either the excitatory callosal hypotheses or the diffuse inhibitory hypothesis. Alone, neither hypothesis suggests anything other than left hemispheric superiority for all linguistic chores. When the stimulus is presented to the left hemisphere, the grapheme would be recognized (in a fixed, low percentage of trials in the Regard and Landis study) and then translated into a corresponding phoneme in 'association' cortex, and finally transmitted to frontal cortex for encoding as speech. The excitatory hypothesis might suggest some degradation of the signal during interhemispheric transfer, but certainly not increased semantic processing, and the diffuse inhibitory hypothesis offers no possibilities for right hemispheric superiority here.

The topographical inhibitory hypothesis, however, postulates a specific callosal transfer mechanism that might be involved. That is, unlike the entire *intra*hemispheric process of stimulus decoding, the inhibitory *inter*hemispheric transfer required to send the right hemisphere's response to the speech mechanisms of the left hemisphere would result in a qualitative change in the information of the hemispheres. Given some kind of 'semantic network' organization of the appropriate cortex (rather than a dictionary-like grapheme- or morpheme-

Left Hemisphere   Right Hemisphere

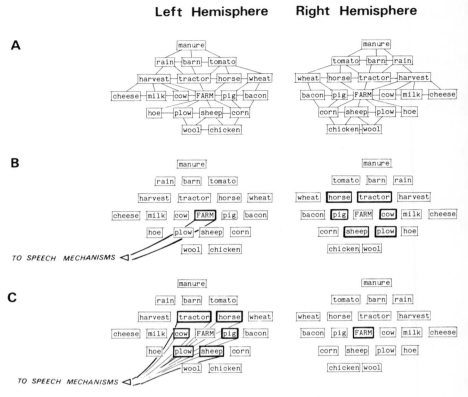

Figure 4.1 A portion of a possible 'agricultural' semantic network. A complex system of associations would exist among these and related words with agricultural meanings. In A, the bilateral network is shown. In B, when a portion of the semantic network (the stimulus, 'farm') is activated on the left, it is translated directly to speech-related motor activity. In C, when the same portion of the semantic network ('farm') is activated on the right, translation into speech requires at least one callosal transfer. If inhibitory, the perceived word would be suppressed and words with close semantic content would be activated for translation into speech.

network), inhibition of one element in the semantic network would mean its suppression *together with the activation of semantically related elements* in the network. The interhemispheric implications of this mechanism are then of interest.

As illustrated in figure 4.1, bilaterally similar semantic networks would decode test stimuli in similar fashion, but the right hemisphere has the additional chore of sending its response to the left hemisphere speech mechanisms. An inhibitory transfer would suppress the correct response and facilitate semantically related, but incorrect, possibilities for the left hemisphere to offer as responses. In other words, working through the left hemisphere, the right hemisphere would be expected to produce semantic paralexia-like responses. In contrast, although the left hemisphere would likely have the same effect on the right hemisphere, the left hemisphere's verbal response would not require the (inhibitory) callosal transfer of its information to the right, and would consequently show no tendency for semantic paralexia. The stimulus perceived at the posterior left cortex would be transmitted (over excitatory routes) to the left frontal cortex for speech output.

Regard and Landis themselves explained their results in terms of the inherent capabilities of the cerebral hemispheres, but it is apparent that the cognitive 'asymmetry' might be the result of the 'asymmetry' of callosal activity (the need for the right hemisphere to express itself through the left, but not vice versa). It should be mentioned at this point that, although the right hemisphere is unquestionably inferior at (and in the normal brain perhaps totally incapable of) vocal expression, Zaidel's studies of the split-brain patients (1976, 1978, 1979) leave no doubt that the right hemisphere in those patients is capable of reasonably good language comprehension (said to be comparable to that of a normal 11-year-old child). Although the right hemisphere may not normally be able to *utilize* its semantic network in overt behavioral ways, some such network is likely to exist and an inhibitory corpus callosum would allow for some interesting interactions between two similar networks.

The number of studies on hemispheric studies which can be reinterpreted *post hoc* in this way is probably quite large. Although suggestive of what the corpus callosum normally does, greater certainty that we are dealing with specifically callosal functions can be obtained in studies on patients with limited brain damage.

Indications of callosal functions in abnormal brains

One of the principal methods of neuropsychological research is to test patients with known brain damage and to infer the normal functions of that part of the brain from what the patient cannot do. Such a research technique has until recently been inappropriate for determining the functions of small brain regions – since the precise location of brain damage was unlikely to be known until autopsy, but it remains one of the most fruitful research methods for deducing the functions which normally occur in relatively large regions of the brain.

The importance of clinical neuropsychology in evaluating the relative contributions of large portions of the brain cannot be doubted and particularly for the *first* question of the localization of brain function – i.e. localization to one or the other of the cerebral hemispheres – neurological signs and symptoms and non-invasive measures of cerebral function are normally sufficient to identify the side of the bleeding or tumor. Comparisons between, for example, left and right frontal damage, or left temporal and left parietal damage can therefore be made and conclusions drawn concerning the functions of large portions of the brain.

For laterality research, there are three principal conditions which shed light on hemisphere functions and the role of the corpus callosum. These are: (i) unilateral brain damage – usually trauma (such as gun wounds) or unilateral intracranial hemorrhage (usually following the rupture of a cerebral aneurysm, where the brain is damaged by the forceful release of blood from a major artery in the brain); (ii) agenesis of the corpus callosum (a relatively rare condition in which the corpus callosum alone or the corpus callosum and anterior commissure do not develop in a brain which is sometimes otherwise fairly normal); and (iii) callosumotomy or surgical transection of the corpus callosum (performed either during the excision of a tumor lying somewhere along the midline of the brain or performed to prevent the spread of epileptic foci to the contralateral hemisphere).

Unilateral brain damage

The principal interest of the topographical inhibitory hypothesis is that it implies a role for the right hemisphere which accords with recent work on brain-damaged patients, suggesting a 'contextual' or 'framework-building' role of the normal right hemisphere.

In a series of studies comparing the cognitive capabilities of left- or right-hemisphere-damaged patients, Gardner and associates have focused on the high-level talents of the right-hemisphere when the left hemisphere is incapacitated. Rather than examine the experimentally tractable, but psychologically less interesting lateral differences in the cognition of nonsense syllables, tonal discrimination and reaction times, they have attempted to evaluate the right hemisphere's contribution to characteristically high-level cognition.

In early papers Gardner and Denes (1973) and Gardner et al. (1975) reported that right-hemisphere damage results in anomalous affect and an inability to understand non-verbal cartoons. From the reactions of right-hemisphere-damaged patients to non-verbal cartoons, they concluded that 'the left hemisphere[-damaged] patient tends to exhibit those preferences and reactions of a normal individual deprived of linguistic output . . . ; the right hemisphere[-damaged] patient resembles a 'sophisticated language machine' responding appropriately to linguistic messages, but with a tendency to extrapolate illegitimately on the basis of fragmentary data.' Despite the inability to communicate verbally, the individual with an abnormal left hemisphere, but a normal right hemisphere could appreciate the comical nature of the cartoons. Surprisingly, however, the individual with only a normal left hemisphere would often 'miss the point' of the cartoons. Although fully capable of describing in words the elements of the cartoon, frequently those elements could not be pieced together into the coherent humorous whole.

Related findings were obtained by Brownell *et al.* (1983). They tested twelve patients with right-hemisphere damage on their ability to choose a humorous ending to a verbal joke from among four alternatives. For example, the body of one such joke was as follows

The neighborhood borrower approached Mr Smith on Sunday after-noon and inquired: 'Say Smith, are you using your lawnmower this afternoon?'
'Yes, I am,' Smith replied warily.
The neighborhood borrower then answered: . . .

And the patients had to choose the most appropriate ending:

Ending No. 1 (correct): 'Fine, then you won't be needing your golf clubs, I'll just borrow them.'
Ending No. 2 (non-sequitur): 'You know, the grass is greener on the other side.'
Ending No. 3 (straightforward, neutral): 'Do you think I could use it when you are done?'
Ending No. 4 (straightforward, sad): 'Gee, if only I had enough money, I could buy my own.'

Not surprisingly they found that (i) the right-hemisphere-damaged patients simply could not choose the humorous ending as often as control subjects. More interestingly, however, they also found that (ii) the right-hemisphere-damaged patients preferred the *non-sequitur* ending more than the controls. Brownell *et al.* interpreted the latter finding as indicating a *normal* predilection for the *surprise* element in humor, but a clearly abnormal inability in 'integrating the content across parts of the narrative.' The results appear to support a two-element model of humor, requiring the ability to detect surprise and the ability to establish coherence – capabilities which were dissociated in their right-hemisphere-damaged patients. In the present context, however, it is of greater interest that they found a high-level cognitive deficit – the inability to construct a coherent whole from appropriate verbal elements.

In a subsequent study Winner and Gardner (1977) demonstrated that comprehension of metaphors also requires an intact right hemisphere. 'The difficulties displayed by the patients with right hemisphere lesions in matching metaphors with pictures, along with their unquestioned acceptance of the literal depictions . . . , indicates that an intact left hemisphere does not of itself ensure adequate comprehension of all linguistic messages.' While 'the left hemisphere appears crucial for full appreciation of the denotation of words . . . , the right hemisphere is necessary for the acceptance of connotative language . . . , the detec-tion of absurd or humorous content . . . , and the mapping of figurative language on to situations in which it is appropriate.' Again, an intact and functional left hemisphere – far from proving itself to be the sole interpreter at an abstract conceptual level – proved to be hopelessly literal and without insight into the underlying meaning of metaphors.

In a more recent attempt to separate the cognitive and affective contributions of the hemispheres, Wapner et al. (1981) tested similar patients on their abilities to assess the plausibility of story elements, to select appropriate punch lines for jokes and to integrate elements of a story into a coherent narrative. They concluded that right-hemisphere-damaged patients 'exhibit a striking amount of difficulty in handling complex linguistic materials.' 'While the ability to remember isolated details and wordings is often preserved, they have clear difficulties in integrating specific information, in drawing proper inferences and morals, and in assessing the appropriateness of various facts, situations and characterizations.' Although the ability to use words and speech itself are normal, 'they often lack a full understanding of the context of an utterance, the presuppositions entailed or the tone of the conversational exchange.'

Pursuing the high-level cognitive capabilities of the right hemisphere, Brownell et al. (1984) examined the effects of unilateral brain damage on the comprehension of words. Specifically they had left- or right-hemisphere-damaged patients classify common adjectives according to their semantic 'similarity.' The adjectives (warm, cold, deep, shallow, loving, hateful, wise and foolish) were presented in groups of three and the patients selected the two which 'go together.' For example, 'deep' and 'shallow' are antonyms, whereas 'deep' and 'wise' are metaphorically similar. Likewise, 'cold' and 'warm' are denotative antonyms, but 'loving' and 'warm' are metaphorically related. None of the patients was incapable of the task, but they classified the words in ways different from each other and different from the controls. Specifically the patients with right-hemisphere damage 'relied more on denotative meaning relations (e.g., antonymic similarity); patients with left-hemisphere pathology relied more on meaning relations based on connotation (e.g., metaphoric equivalence); and normal controls used relations representing both classes of meaning components.' Brownell et al. (1984) concluded that:

> The picture of understanding obtained in the present study indicates that, even at the single word level, certain aspects of the meaning of emotional language may be lost to right hemisphere [-damaged] patients – specifically, those having to do with connotations rather than sheer denotation.

Viewing the patients with right-sided damage as people with only a functional left hemisphere, it would seem that the role of the left hemisphere is denotative and literal, while that of the right hemisphere is more conceptual. Patients with only a functional right hemisphere tend to be able to grasp the overall picture, but have trouble with explicit linguistic manipulations. Gardner et al. (1983) conclude:

These patients seem to have impaired access to certain bits of denotative linguistic knowledge, whether this knowledge be at the level of single words or at the level of sentences. They therefore fall back on types of knowledge – either the connotative elements of word meaning or the gist of a conversation – that are not so tightly bound to the left hemisphere language system, but that rest on more general, lexical, conceptual or interpretive cognitive apparatus.

Related conclusions concerning the cognitive capabilities of the right hemisphere have been reached by others. Caramazza *et al.* (1976) found that right-hemisphere-damaged patients had no difficulty in responding to: 'John is taller than Bill. Who is taller?' But a relatively simple transformation to: 'John is taller than Bill. Who is shorter?' produced significant errors. That is to say as long as *literal* manipulations of the wording could produce correct responses, there was no problem, but when the relationship required conceptualization, the literal left hemisphere ran into trouble. Despite a degree of linguistic competence, 'understanding' – as we normally understand it! – was lacking.

Previously Zurif *et al.* (1974) found that left-hemisphere damage resulted in the classification of words by their connotations rather than denotations. For example, rather than group trout and shark together as types of fish, they would put tiger and shark together as examples of fierceness. Such results indicate that denotation is a function of the left hemisphere and connotation that of the right.

Cavalli *et al.* (1981) found that right-hemisphere damage had no effects upon simple 'traditional' linguistic tests, but sentence construction from a vertically presented list of several words was significantly impaired. 'The most common type of error was to leave the sentence unfinished or to produce sentences with unlikely meanings' – that is grammatically correct but conceptually anomalous. It is indicative of the lack of depth of 'traditional' tests (defining words, matching adjectives with nouns, antonyms and synonyms) that the brain-damaged patients performed normally on them, while a seemingly simple task of producing a meaningful sentence proved difficult. The inability to rearrange words which remain in sight at all times indicates that the right-hemisphere-damaged patients were not suffering simply from a memory deficit. This was also the case in a similar study done by Gardner *et al.* (1983) in which sentences written on individual cards required sequential ordering to produce a coherent narrative. Although the patients with right-sided damage were capable of everyday linguistic processing, when asked to produce such narratives, they performed no better than *aphasic* patients with damage to the so-called 'language' left hemisphere.

Is it any surprise that the mental symptoms of brain damage are sometimes overlooked, if the traditional linguistic tests are geared to such a low level of understanding that questions of 'meaning' beyond the literal are not raised? It would probably be unfair to blame the busy clinician for failing to detect right-hemisphere talents, but these recent findings of subtle, but consistently noted deficits of language following right-sided damage certainly suggest that we should not rely too heavily on perfunctory clinical examinations when it comes to constructing a theory of brain function.

Gainotti and colleagues have also pursued the question of what specific language deficits are found in right-hemisphere-damaged patients. Their first study on this topic was a replication of work reported by Lesser (1974), who had found that right-sided damage left the patients with a normal ability to process phonological and syntactical information, but with a significantly lower capacity to make so-called semantic lexical discriminations. For example, when individual concrete nouns were read aloud (for example, 'house') by the investigators, the right-hemisphere-damaged patients showed a significant tendency to choose pictures of incorrect but semantically related items (such as 'church'), but not pictures of phonemically related items (such as 'mouse'). While improving on the mode of presentation (to avoid possible influences of left visual field neglect), they found essentially the same effect as that reported previously by others. Moreover, the same effect was still apparent when the influences of a general mental deterioration, often seen in such patients, was controlled for (these experiments are summarized in Gainotti et al., 1983).

In their next study they investigated the possibility of visuospatial disturbances (as distinct from neglect of a half-field) having influenced the apparent deficits in semantic processing. This was accomplished by classifying all errors as semantic, visuospatial or both (visuosemantic). For example, if, in response to 'apple,' the patient pointed to a picture of a 'ball,' this was scored as a 'visuospatial' error. If the patient pointed to 'pear,' this was scored as a 'semantic' error, whereas selection of a 'peach' would be a 'visuosemantic' error.

It is noteworthy that the conventional 'visuospatial' characterization of the right hemisphere would certainly predict that the problems which these patients encounter should be due to the loss of the capacity to *visualize* internally the spatial qualities of the spoken words. To the contrary what Gainotti and colleagues (1983) found was that:

> these patients produce mainly visual-semantic and purely semantic errors and that only a relatively small number of their wrong responses can be classified as purely visual. . . . These findings clearly argue against the hypothesis that semantic discrimination errors of right-brain-damaged patients may be due to a purely visuoperceptual disorder and rather point to the existence in these patients of a true semantic-lexical impairment. (p. 162)

They are cautious about how definitive such results can be, given uncertainty about the actual brain pathology, but they point out that their findings on such patients provide a

> mirror image of the linguistic capabilities described as characteristic of the intact right hemisphere. In fact, data obtained in split-brain patients (Zaidel, 1976, 1978) and in subjects submitted after childhood to a left ('dominant') hemispherectomy (Smith, 1966; Gott, 1973; Burklund and Smith, 1977) have consistently shown that the *intact right hemisphere* (a) possesses a high capability to understand the meaning of single words, (b) performs very poorly on tasks requiring phonemic analysis, and (c) has an auditory lexicon that is richer than its visual lexicon. Conversely, results of the investigations reported here have shown that *right-brain-damaged patients*: (a) score significantly worse than normal controls on various tasks of semantic–lexical discrimination even when the influence of associated variables (such as unilateral spatial neglect or general cognitive impairment) is ruled out; (b) do not perform worse than normal controls when the number of phonemic errors obtained on two different tests of word comprehension and of nonsense syllables discrimination is taken into account; (c) tend to commit a higher number of semantic errors when the lexical representation is accessed through the auditory modality than when it is accessed through the visual (reading) modality.

They conclude by stating that the results of their investigations 'consistently show that right hemisphere lesions produce a selective disorder of the semantic level of language.'

Approaching the question of the high-level functions of the right hemisphere from a slightly different angle, there has been a recent surge of interest in the emotional capacities of the 'non-dominant' hemisphere. Findings which have been interpreted in terms of the 'affective' role of the right hemisphere (Tucker, 1981) have been reported by Ross and Mesulam (1979) and Heilman *et al.* (1975). Ross and Mesulam (1979) found that the production of propositional language production was intact following lesions to the anterior right hemisphere, but there were deficits in the ability to express the affective and connotative aspects of language. Conversely Heilman *et al.* (1975) found that, after posterior right-hemisphere damage, literal understanding of the spoken word was normal, but the 'understanding' was unusually shallow with the affective implications of language not properly appreciated.

It is worth emphasizing that, in conversations among people without brain-damage, it would be entirely normal to ask someone whether or not he in fact *understood* what had just been said if he failed to exhibit the appropriate emotional response to affect-laden words or used affect-laden phrases in a matter-of-fact monotone voice. Although it is the lack of emotion which is the manifest *behavioral* anomaly of such patients, it must be asked whether or not normal *cognitive* processing, as distinct from the emotive implications, has indeed taken place. My suspicion is that the *loss of emotion* in many right-hemisphere-damaged patients is but one particularly obvious aspect of the failure to appreciate the cognitive implications of language. At the level of the central nervous system, it may be primarily a deficit in information-processing, and only secondarily a matter of abnormal inactivity of the limbic system (or autonomic nervous system, etc.) in the failure to express emotions.

One of the most interesting recent developments in the neuropsychology of the cerebral hemispheres is the finding of deficits of 'attention' (as distinct from unilateral neglect) in patients with right-hemisphere damage. Although speech production and, at a literal level, speech comprehension are normal, right-sided damage often results in the inability to 'concentrate' on a given task, in the 'wandering' of the mind and in a resultant mixing together of apparently unrelated ideas.

A state in which various deficits of attention are found has been characterized by Geschwind (1982) as a 'confusional state' – which he believes is the *most* frequently encountered psychic disturbance in the neurological clinic. Such patients show one or several of the following disturbances: (i) loss of coherence, (ii) paramnesia (*incorrect* recollection, as distinct from failure to recollect), (iii) paraphasia (incorrect speaking with word substitution and jumbling of phrases which make speech unintelligible, but not the inability to speak), (iv) jargon production, (v) inattention to environmental stimuli, (vi) disturbances of writing, (vii) denial of illness and (viii) playful behavior. Such a list appears at first glance to be a grab-bag of minor disturbances, but seven of the eight can be interpreted as the loss or rapid dissolution of the overall context of ongoing language processes (table 4.1). As a result the intact and functional left hemisphere becomes 'confused,' as the implications and normal conceptual framework of one's own language and that of other's repeatedly slips away.

Geschwind's view of the right hemisphere's role in attention is still considered unconventional – at least partly due to the fact that the word 'attention' is normally used in reference to the cortical arousal effects of the *brainstem*. Without challenging the content of his arguments, I would argue that he has focused on an extremely important feature of the right hemisphere, but has chosen the wrong label. Not only is 'attention' normally associated with the level of brainstem arousal effects, but also it is associated with the human will – which no one would want to suggest is resident in one hemisphere only. Parenthetically it is worth noting that Geschwind did not in fact interpret right hemisphere functions and specifically the confusional states in terms of callosal activity. On the one hand, he might have been naturally attracted to this 'connectionist' view of hemispheric specializations due to his longstanding advocacy of connectionism (Geschwind, 1965), but, on the other hand, his work on anatomical cerebral asymmetries has lent crucial support to the reductionist view that the hemispheres differ because of asymmetrical cortical 'modules' (Geschwind and Levitsky, 1968).

The ability to 'attend' to relevant stimuli may be an important result of intact functioning of the right hemisphere, but perhaps there is a more accurate label to summarize this mode of cognitive processing which is as characteristic of the right hemisphere as language is of the left hemisphere. Geschwind's own description of the deficits of right hemisphere damage does not require the use of the 'attention' label and indeed he describes the clinical condition as one of 'confusion' rather than one of 'inattention.' If right hemisphere dysfunction (whether due to organic lesions or relatively mild metabolic deficits which have asymmetric effects) can lead to a state of confusion, then the appropriate label for the *normal* contribution of the right hemisphere might be something along the lines of 'framework-building.' In other words, being 'unconfused' is not really the same thing as being 'attentive;' it would seem more accurate to describe the unconfused state as capable of remaining 'within the appropriate context' of ongoing thoughts or conversation. The presence or absence of the confusional state may therefore be said to be due to the absence or presence of the overall cognitive framework – regardless of the amount of brainstem arousal or the amount of 'effort' made by the subject to attend to relevant stimuli.

The only clear advantage of the 'attention' and 'inattention' labels is their relationship with the phenomenon of unilateral neglect, which is known to be more severe following right than left hemisphere damage. Mesulam (1981) among others has argued that there is a mechanism for bilateral attention in the right hemisphere of man and has shown that the clinical evidence is almost as convincing as that for language functions in the left. The evidence for this 'attentional' involvement of the right hemisphere comes primarily from a comparison of the effects of left and right hemisphere damage. When stroke, trauma or tumor affects the left parietal lobe, patients will often show language deficits, but will normally continue to respond to visual stimuli in both the left and right visual fields. In contrast, comparable right-sided damage will far more frequently produce unilateral neglect – often a complete inattention to visual stimuli to the left of the midline. This abnormality can extend to both auditory and somesthetic stimuli, but is most common and dramatic when patients are asked to make simple drawings (see, for example, figure 4.2). In extreme cases all of the environment on the left will be ignored, although these deficits usually recover over the ensuing weeks.

Interestingly there is a comparable neglect of body space – often manifest in the failure to shave the left half of the face. Associated neurological deficits on the left (paresis, etc.) may not merely be ignored, they may be actively denied or explained away with bizarre excuses and rationalizations. Such 'confabulation' indicates that the

Table 4.1 A comparison of the excitatory and inhibitory theories of callosal function

→	Excitatory callosal hypothesis	Inhibitory callosal hypothesis	Current empirical findings
Normal	Hemispheric asymmetries due to inherent anatomical and neurotransmitter hemispheric asymmetries. The corpus callosum serves, if at all, to reduce hemispheric specializations.	Hemispheric asymmetries due primarily to callosal effects. The corpus callosum serves to augment hemispheric differences already present due to morphological differences.	Anatomical and neurotransmitter asymmetries have been found,[1] but correlations between such asymmetries and behavioral asymmetries are weak[2] or are contrary to predictions.[3]
Callosal agenesis	Total agenesis would leave hemispheric specializations intact due to morphological asymmetries. The development of paracallosal interhemispheric communication is the only factor which would distinguish these patients from the callosumectomy patients. Due to decreased interhemispheric cross-talk, there would be increased functional asymmetry.	Total agenesis would prevent the development of hemispheric specializations otherwise due to callosal effects. Only language dominance would be expected due to the normal hemispheric competition for midline speech organs, but non-language specializations would not be found. Compared with normals, there would be reduced hemispheric asymmetry. Compared with callosumectomy patients, there would be decreased functional asymmetry.	Agenesis patients do not show the disconnection syndrome.[4] Increased bilateralization has been reported,[5] but the evidence remains inconclusive.

Callosumectomy	Callosumectomy would prevent the 'leakage' of specializations to the contralateral side, i.e. prevent bilateralization, of normally asymmetric functions. Postoperative augmentation of differential specializations predicted.	Callosumectomy would prevent the further development of hemispheric asymmetries. The duration of the preoperative state would determine the degree of lateral specialization and the duration of the postoperative state would determine the degree of subsequent bilateralization. Continuing reduction in postoperative asymmetries predicted.	Postoperative gradual bilateralization of function found, particularly increases in the verbal capacities of the right hemisphere.[6]
Right-hemisphere damage	Specific language deficits which are unrelated to visuospatial deficits are not predicted.	Deficits in the understanding of the context and connotations of language are predicted.	Deficits in the understanding of context found (see text).

Notes: 1. Rubens (1977). 2. Whitaker and Ojemann (1977) and Walker (1980). 3. Galaburda (1984). 4. Milner and Jeeves (1979). 5. Sperry (1969). 6. Gazzaniga *et al.* (1979).

MODEL   RH LESION

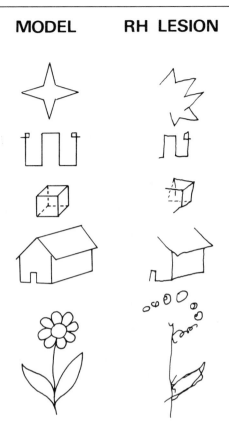

Figure 4.2 Drawings by patients after having suffered right-sided brain damage. Neglect of the left-hand side of space is apparent both in spontaneous drawings and those made following a model.

intact left hemisphere is reluctant to acknowledge that the mute right hemisphere is having any difficulties, but what is most surprising is that when the left hemipshere suffers damage the right hemisphere does not show similar unilateral neglect. Unlike the intact but isolated left hemisphere (or either hemisphere in other species), the human right hemisphere has a good understanding of *bilateral* corporeal and extracorporeal space.

Within the present context the crucial question is whether the notable asymmetry of such brain damage (in man) is due to asymmetries of attention itself or asymmetries in the conceptualization of objects and events within their proper contexts. Particularly in attending to objects in the left half of the visual field, the bilateral nature of right-hemisphere perception is clear indication that the scope of right-hemispheric perception is particularly wide, but again it may be that the core talent of the right hemisphere is its capacity for extracting the context and viewing the perceptual (and conceptual) field as a whole. Rather than the narrow and literal focus of the left hemisphere, the right hemisphere may be inclined to view extracorporeal space, corporeal space and, most importantly, 'linguistic space' in terms of its overall meaning.

Kinsbourne's (1978) alternative explanation of unilateral neglect, however, deserves consideration. He has argued that, since the patient is required by the doctor in the hospital setting to communicate using the language capacities of the left hemisphere, an asymmetric activation of the cerebral hemispheres could result in an aggravation of left-sided (right-hemispheric) neglect and the amelioration of right-sided (left-hemispheric) neglect. The unilateral neglect which is more severe following right-hemisphere damage might therefore not reflect a gross asymmetry of 'attentional capacities,' so much as asymmetrical activation. At any rate according to Geschwind (1982) the confusional states are – if less dramatic and less easily illustrated in neurology texts – more frequently encountered following right-sided damage than the specific, transitory inattention to contralateral environmental stimuli.

Finally it is noteworthy that, in both man and monkeys, callosumotomy will produce a transient unilateral neglect in either an intact human left hemisphere or in either hemisphere contralateral to appropriate cortical damage. While questions remain concerning the mechanisms of recovery and the postoperative organization of the perceptual system, the disruption due to callosal section is direct evidence supporting the idea that the bilateral 'attention' of the right hemisphere is due to normal callosal mechanisms.

SURGICAL SECTION OF THE CORPUS CALLOSUM

Although a lesion of an entirely different nature, severance of the corpus callosum would eliminate the right hemisphere's contextual role as effectively as right-hemisphere damage. Although the right hemisphere nonetheless receives its normal dose of sensory stimulation, it would no longer receive the selective patterns of inhibition from the left hemisphere and no longer contribute its somewhat different linguistic experiences to the speech activities of the left. Subtle cognitive deficits similar to those of right-hemisphere damage would therefore be predicted in the split-brain patients (table 4.2) – specifically a deficit in understanding the contextual and connotative implications of language, simultaneously with the garrulousness and punning typical of patients with right-hemisphere damage. Indeed frequent remarks have been made concerning the unusual conversation of the split-brain patients. Sperry (1968) has stated explicitly: 'I want to caution against an impression that these patients are better off mentally without their cerebral commissures. . . . Their intellect is . . . handicapped in ways that are probably not revealed in the ordinary tests.' He also notes 'deficits in the ability to grasp broad, long-term or distant implications

Table 4.2 Eight features of the 'confusional states' which are commonly produced by right-hemisphere disorders, and their interpretation in terms of a mirror-image negative relationship between the cerebral hemispheres

Clinical features	Geschwind's (1982) definitions	Interpretation in terms of the inability to produce a mirror-image negative pattern in the right hemisphere via the corpus callosum
Loss of coherence	Failure to 'pay attention;' abrupt shifts in the topic of conversation; disruption of the overall pattern of action despite the correct performance of fragments ('ideational-apraxia-like').	Context of ongoing internal or external speech not apprehended; speech shifts with literal meanings of words, inappropriate to overall direction of the conversation; competent use of unilaterally stored motor information, but actions performed out of their proper context.
Paramnesia	Distortion rather than loss of memory. Information is available, but misplaced and jumbled with incorrect ideas.	Correct datum placed within bizarre contexts as a consequence of the loss of automatically generated right-hemisphere context. Distortions through literal punning.
Wild paraphasias and propagation of error	Once an error is made, other items in the environment are brought into apparent coherence with the error.	Literal left-hemispheric extrapolation from both correct and incorrect data because of the inability to access right-hemisphere context.
Occupational jargon	Use of stilted language reminiscent of official documents.	Exclusive use of left-hemispheric denotative language.

Inattention to environmental cues	Failure to use environmental information.	Inability to access 'contextual' perceptual information; persistent reliance on left-sided language(?).
Isolated or predominant disturbance of writing	Dissolution of writing; spatially abnormal, incorrect words, misspellings.	Incorrect words and misspellings a consequence of the inability to maintain the context of the ongoing sentence over the prolonged time periods required to write language on paper.
Unconcern or denial of illness	Denial of illness or lack of concern about it.	Inability to appreciate the full implications of the present illness.
Apparently playful behavior	Funny and witty remarks; non-deliberate facetiousness; unintentional collocation of ideas.	Garrulousness and punning due to persistence of left-hemispheric literal language process, unconstrained by normal conceptual boundaries.

of a situation' and that 'their conversation tends to be restricted mainly to what is immediate and simple' (Sperry, 1974).

Dimond (1979a) has made similar comments about the unusual conversation of the split-brain patients, but was particularly struck by the inappropriate nature of their emotional expression. He has noted that one young patient related the news of his mother's severe illness and impending death in a conversational voice which revealed none of the usual unhappy emotions. He related the news as 'something funny' that had happened, and treated the topic as humorous. Both Dimond and, more recently, Flor-Henry (1983) have interpreted these findings as indicating fundamentally different emotional orientations of the cerebral hemispheres, but again we must ask how such a dichotomy could arise. If one hemisphere processes information and reaches happy and optimistic conclusions, whereas the other hemisphere takes essentially the same information and reaches sad and pessimistic conclusions, it could be that either (i) major hemispheric asymmetries exist, *or* (ii) the nature of the interhemispheric communication affects their cognitive processing. Flor-Henry has argued that the asymmetry is likely to be at the level of brainstem neurotransmitters. Since drugs known to have facilitating and inhibiting effects on neurotransmitters can have major effects on mood, it would suffice to have excess serotonin in the left hemisphere and acetylcholine in the right to produce hemispheres with slightly different affective orientations. The pharmacological implications of a brainstem asymmetry are of course appealing to the clinician, but currently the alternative view of the causal mechanisms involved seems equally viable. That is callosal activity could produce hemispheres with different degrees of connotative development of language, and the neurotransmitter asymmetries could be a result of them.

Flor-Henry (1983) goes on to explain various features of schizophrenia and manic-depression and even sex differences in terms of such an asymmetry and its disturbances, but the alternative approach appears to lead to similar conclusions. That is if prior to the expression of emotions there is an asymmetry of high-level cognition such that the left hemisphere is continually involved in the literal decoding of language, while the right hemisphere is continually processing the context and implications of language, then it would invariably be the right hemisphere which understands the emotional content of language, while the left hemisphere revolves in the world of literal meanings (and, by inference, the lighter emotions involved in puns and verbal quips without most of their cognitive implications). Functional differences between the cerebral hemispheres and tonic differences in neurotransmitters would then be a consequence of a high-level cognitive asymmetry which itself is a function of callosal activity.

Brief discussion of psychopathological states is made in chapter 7, but is far too complex an issue to pursue here. Suffice it to say that the 'contextual' role of the right hemisphere which has been identified in patients with brain damage suggests that many of the abnormalities of emotion seen both in brain-damaged patients and in psychopathological conditions may be a *consequence* of abnormal cognitive functioning within the right hemisphere rather than abnormalities of emotion *per se*. In any event the split-brain patients exhibit mild abnormalities of both thought and emotion, which can be plausibly related to a dissociation between literal verbal thinking and its larger conceptual framework.

In spite of the fact that the split-brain patients can be experimentally 'tricked' into having hemispheres with contradictory information, Sperry's description of the mental condition of the split-brain patients is quite different from the 'two-personalities in one skull' characterization which seems to predominate in the popular media. Instead of two more-or-less complete 'selves,' it would seem that, in terms of the postoperative personality, commissurotomy produces one somewhat *incomplete* self – capable of getting around in everyday life, but showing deficits in characteristically *human* cognition if indeed the 'broad,' 'long-term' and 'distant' implications slip by. Somehow in the welter of split-brain research and supported by the neurosurgeon's insistence that his patients are 'ordinary,' the subtle but repeatedly noted cognitive abnormalities of the split-brain patients have not been rigorously studied.

Unlike those individuals who are born without a corpus callosum (discussed on pp. 142–3), the split-brain patients have experienced many years during which most callosal functions were normal. Consequently their right hemispheres are thought likely to have developed the specializations typical of the normal brain, whereas those of the complete agenesis patients should have right hemispheres which are *abnormal in not having received the psychological effects of normal callosal activity*. The split-brain patients, however, should not have the normal mechanisms for *accessing* right-hemisphere talents through the corpus callosum. They are therefore predicted to have rather *normal* hemispheric lateralization (whether or not the corpus callosum plays a role in the development of bilateral asymmetries), but rather *abnormal* behavior due to a failure to make use of, in particular, the contextual and connotative aspects of right-hemisphere linguistic processing. In contrast, the agenesis patients are expected to have somewhat abnormal hemispheric specializations (specifically lacking the specializations of the right hemisphere; see pp. 142–3), but due to the inherent plasticity of the developing brain, their behavior may be more normal – specifically connotatively and contextually intact – than the split-brain patients.

The main difference between the split-brain and the acallosal patients lies in the usage of the right hemisphere. The split-brain patients would have a storehouse of essentially normal right-hemisphere talents which cannot be accessed over normal callosal routes. The acallosal patient would lack this unique, complementary neural system, but would therefore not suffer from the inability to access it. The missing right hemisphere talents would likely produce a lowered intelligence, but not bizarre dissociation between thought and affect or language and context.

Barring other kinds of neurological abnormalities in the split-brain patients, it would be expected that callosal section would be far less debilitating than right-hemisphere damage – where an entire cognitive system becomes totally dysfunctional. Particularly insofar as non-callosal routes exist for accessing the right hemisphere (the 'vertical' aspect of right-hemisphere functioning), use of right-hemisphere talents may yet be possible. Nonetheless insofar as left-hemisphere language can no longer generate or access contextual information directly from the right hemisphere, a tendency toward 'literalness' and a failure to grasp implications which are obvious to the normal individual would be predicted. As yet the split-brain patients have not been studied with an eye specifically to such cognitive deficits.

Theoretically the split-brain patients provide the best testing-ground for the hypotheses on callosal function. If the corpus callosum plays a role predominantly in brain development (and not in adulthood), its transection in adulthood should be virtually without *cognitive* effects. On the other hand, if the corpus callosum is involved in 'accessing' information from the contralateral hemisphere (by whatever mechanism), then its loss should produce notable, high-level symptoms.

Until ten years ago the bulk of evidence seemed to favor the view that specifically cognitive deficits were few, mild or absent, but the negative view is no longer dominant for two reasons: (i) Most of the *sensory and motor* deficits following callosal section have been discovered only with the new generation of experimental techniques, developed by Sperry and colleagues. Moreover, (ii) virtually all of the high-level cognitive (and specifically language-related) talents of the right hemisphere have been discovered only in the last ten to fifteen years, and made possible by a combination of more sophisticated diagnostic techniques to ascertain the location of brain damage prior to autopsy *and*, importantly, a much more subtle understanding of human cognition – specifically the role of 'context' in making sense out of literal language.

While the clinician may of necessity be interested in only a superficial understanding of the patient's psychic state ('What is your name? Where are you now?'), cognitive psychologists, linguists and those working in artificial intelligence are very much aware of the hierarchical complexities of language comprehension in particular, and of the fact that some aspects of cognitive systems can become damaged, while others remain intact. For these reasons the bulk of the negative evidence from several decades ago concerning the role of the corpus callosum in cognition simply cannot be taken seriously.

Still it must be admitted that the reported 'ordinariness' of the split-brain patients presents a problem for this perspective on callosal functions. It may be the case – as sometimes argued – that there are simply too many uncontrolled factors and too great a diversity of outcome following callosal transection to allow for unambiguous evaluation of the psychological effects of callosal transection. Specifically (i) there is a wide variety of symptoms following callosal transection (varying from 'ordinariness' to total and permanent aphasia); (ii) various commissural structures, including the anterior commissure, thalamic adhesion and the hippocampal commissure, have been cut in some patients; and (iii) there is a variety of extra-callosal damage as a result of prolonged epilepsy. These factors may simply preclude the possibility of making any generalizations at all concerning high-level psychological functions of the forebrain commissures. Without implying any sinister motivations, it should also be noted that the neurosurgeons involved in callosal transection are undoubtedly concerned that callosumotomy may someday be viewed as a more harmless version of frontal lobectomy – that is, more destructive than constructive. Granted that major personality changes are not induced by such surgery, clearly the responsible surgeons have a vested interest in viewing their patients as 'ordinary'. High-level psychological, as distinct from perceptual, testing of these patients is still needed.

Clearly the view of the corpus callosum presented in this book suggests that any split-brain patient (who has undergone complete commissurotomy and who has unilateral language capacities but two intact cerebral hemispheres) should show conceptual difficulties similar to those of the right-hemisphere-damaged patients studied by Gardner and colleagues. In contrast to the topographical inhibitory theory of the corpus callosum, the excitatory and diffuse inhibitory theories do not predict high-level cognitive deficits due to callosal section.

An excitatory theory of callosal functions – which implies the approximate duplication of neural information in both hemispheres – would alone predict only minimal effects due to callosal transection. If, however, callosal activity was an important part of an excitatory reverberatory circuit, then it might be argued that callosal excitation would normally allow for the development of the distant implications, connotations, etc., of left-hemispheric language – and conversely that loss of the reverberatory circuit through callosal section would lead to a loss of the connotative (etc.) aspects of language understanding. Such a view of callosal function remains an interesting possible development of the excitatory hypothesis, but the predominantly inhibitory effect of callosal activity appears incongruous within such a hypothesis. At any rate without theoretical amplification of the excitatory hypothesis, callosal transection would not be predicted to have major effects on left-hemispheric language processes.

A diffuse inhibitory model of the corpus callosum predicts a marked decrease in the suppression of contralateral cortex during language activities following callosal transection. As such the development of bilaterally symmetrical capacities of the two hemispheres would seem inevitable. The evidence on this issue is not unambiguous, but there seems to be a consensus that there is increased bilateralization over time of at least language functions (Gazzaniga *et al.*, 1979). Notably right hemispheres which were totally mute following surgery have learned to utilize the left hand for simple linguistic communication. Such post-operative independence of the right hemisphere is conceivably due to the removal of callosal inhibition.

Language deficits – in particular an inability to access the connotations of words – are not an immediate prediction of the diffuse inhibitory hypothesis. Only if the diffuse inhibitory hypothesis were developed to allow for the connotative, metaphorical, contextual (etc.) meanings of words in the right hemisphere would callosal transection then be expected to produce language deficits. Indeed this could be done by simply postulating the existence of appropriate right-sided 'connotation modules' of some kind, but the role of the corpus callosum in this view remains unclear. In other words, insofar as the relationship between denotation and connotation is not explicitly produced via the corpus callosum, callosal section would not be predicted by the diffuse inhibitory hypothesis to result in deficits in the specifically connotative aspects of language.

The topographical inhibitory model predicts both increased bilateralization of functions following the split-brain operation and language deficits essentially identical to those of the right-hemisphere-damaged patients. Specifically in a categorization test similar to that used by Brownell *et al.* (1984) in brain-damaged patients (described on pp. 126–7), the typical left hemisphere strengths of denotation should be favored over the connotative strengths of the right hemisphere. This test remains to be done in the split-brain patients.

AGENESIS OF THE CORPUS CALLOSUM

Absence of the corpus callosum is a relatively rare congenital defect in which the callosal fibers course toward the midline, but terminate in the limbic cortex without crossing to the contralateral hemisphere (figure 4.3). Misplacement of 200 million fibers simply cannot be without effects on brain function, but associated abnormalities have prevented unambiguous identification of the specific role of the corpus callosum. Often other abnormalities, including tumors and microcephaly, are present and hydrocephalus is a common consequence of the agenesis. The remarkable near-normality of some of the agenesis patients, however, suggests that some clues concerning the normal role of the corpus callosum might be found from the study of such patients who do not have other notable brain abnormalities.

Unlike patients who have had the corpus callosum severed after 10–30 years of epileptic but neuroanatomically intact life, those

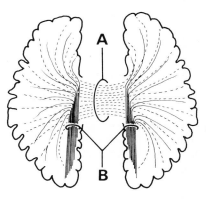

Figure 4.3 The coursing of callosal fibers in the normal brain (dashed lines) and in the brain with 'callosal agenesis' (solid lines) (after Rakic and Yakovlev, 1968). When the callosal fibers terminate on the side where they originate, the so-called bundle of Probst (B) is found, rather than the corpus callosum (A). The bundle courses posteriorly within the cingulate gyrus and terminates in limbic and olfactory cortex. Its functional significance is not known.

individuals who have been born without this tract would never have received whatever cognitive benefits which the corpus callosum bestows. If, as argued above, this commissure allows the 'contextual development' of linguistic messages – and, more generally, generalization of contralateral information – then a congenital deficit of the corpus callosum should surely lead to impaired intelligence. Moreover the cognitive deficits of 'pure' callosal agenesis should not be accompanied by sensory or motor deficits which do not require callosal transfer.

This 'prediction' of the effects of agenesis is of course made *post hoc* – in light of the fact that most such patients are mentally subnormal – often diagnosed as 'idiots' or 'imbeciles,' but sometimes with normal or mildly subnormal intelligence. Chiarello (1980) has calculated a mean verbal IQ of 89 and a mean performance IQ of 89 among the published acallosal cases, but these slightly below average IQs were calculated by excluding all of the retardate cases. Because of the high frequency of other brain abnormalities, it remains empirically an open question whether or not the mental deficits in such patients are a direct result of the loss of this nerve tract.

The predicted relationship between callosal function and intelligence is, however, potentially testable since there are various degrees of callosal agenesis and various degrees of accompanying disorders. The most important variable is the amount of hemispheric communication via the forebrain commissures. The corpus callosum in such cases is not always totally absent and there is often the presence and even compensatory hypertrophy of the anterior commissure. Without more precise knowledge concerning the functional differences between these commissures, it might be assumed that they work in similar fashion, so that intelligence would be a direct function of the number of inter-hemispheric fibers. A factor which must be controlled for, however, is the extent of other morphological abnormalities which can arise in parallel or as a result of the failure of callosal fibers to extend contra-laterally. In practical terms study of the correlation between intelligence and the extent of interhemispheric communication in these patients would be difficult insofar as autopsy would probably be required. Nonetheless the cause of the subnormal intelligence in such cases is of great theoretical interest and diagnostic difficulties may eventually be overcome with PET scans and other means for visualizing the commissures in living subjects.

The various theories of callosal function should be testable in this realm. Unlike an excitatory theory of callosal function, which would not predict a causal link between callosal agenesis and low intelligence, the inhibitory models predict a direct link. Whereas the excitatory theory must explain the low intelligence of such patients in terms of associated brain abnormalities of either a gross morphological, cyto-logical or metabolic kind, the inhibitory theory views the agenesis as primary to the intellectual deficits.

The clinical evidence bearing on this problem is unfortunately incomplete. In a study of thirteen reported cases of callosal agenesis, Selnes (1974) reports that all of the cases with total agenesis were diagnosed as 'idiocy.' In contrast a college student with a normal IQ, reported by Saul and Sperry (1968), showed an enlarged anterior commissure and no cognitive deficits in the tests given.

The mirror-image negative hypothesis clearly implies that the loss of the right hemisphere either through organic lesion or through separa-tion from the left would leave such patients linguistically competent, but functioning without awareness of the full 'paralinguistic' and connotative superstructure which is normally the key to grasping the essential meaning of linguistic messages. Contextual impairments are therefore expected both in the split-brain patients and (to the extent that other commissural fibers have not replaced the missing corpus callosum) also in individuals with callosal agenesis. Semantic paralexias found in normal subjects are predicted *not* to occur in the acallosal subjects.

Summary

As summarized in table 4.2, the topographical excitatory hypothesis alone can explain little of the empirical findings on cerebral laterality. At the very least, the excitatory theory requires consistent anatomical asymmetries to explain asymmetrical functions of the cerebral hemi-spheres. Thus far, the evidence on both anatomical and neurotransmit-ter asymmetries has not shown the extremely high correlation between behavioral and brain asymmetries which the excitatory model requires. Even given much higher correlations of this kind, the actual role of the corpus callosum remains far from clear in such a view. If each hemisphere can be characterized as a collection of specialized 'modules,' why is contralateral input (away from primary sensory areas) of any importance at all, and why should there be steadily increasing contralateral input as we ascend the phylogenetic scale? Perhaps these questions can be answered within the framework of the excitatory hypothesis, but considerable amplification of the excitatory view will be required.

The inhibitory hypotheses, on the other hand, appear to be consistent with the major thrust of the findings concerning lateral specialization and the effects of callosal dysfunction (table 4.2). With the further assumptions required for the topographical inhibitory hypothesis, the inhibitory view of the corpus callosum appears to be consistent with (i) the basic anatomy and physiology of the cortex, and (ii) the major behavioral findings of callosal transection and agenesis. Although explicit demonstration of topographical callosal inhibition at the cellular level has not yet been achieved, the behavioral evidence and physiological plausibility of the hypothesis suggest that a 'mirror-image negative,' as opposed to a 'carbon-copy' relationship between the cerebral hemispheres is possible.

It is worth emphasizing that, insofar as cortical regions communicate via topographical mapping, logically a second area can receive information from a first area in only two ways: either as a 'carbon-copy' replication of a specific configuration of neuronal excitation, or as a 'photographic negative.' Carbon-copy transmission of topographical information is the established rule in relaying sensory information from the sense organs to at least secondary sensory cortical areas – and perhaps beyond, ipsilaterally. Both clinical and experimental studies have indicated that (i) the corpus callosum transfers information between the cerebral cortices, but (ii) not of sufficient strength or appropriate nature always to establish identical engrams bilaterally – as most clearly demonstrated in the unilaterality of human speech. Homotopic callosal inhibition is the first logical alternative mechanism of interhemispheric communication.

Although the idea of callosal *inhibition* has frequently been considered as essential to explain hemispheric specializations (e.g. Kinsbourne, 1974; Denenberg, 1981) and abnormalities of specialization (e.g. Flor-Henry, 1979a) and *mirror-image* transfer via homotopic commissural fibers has been invoked to explain lateral mirror-image confusions in children and animals (e.g. Orton, 1937; Noble, 1968; Corballis and Beale, 1976), the possibility of a *mirror-image negative* relationship has not previously been explored. If, however, the cerebral hemispheres are predominantly symmetrical and connected homotopically, then the mirror-image negative is one of only two possible topographical relationships between them.

In the topographical inhibitory model, the difference between the activity in the left and right hemispheres will be the difference between a focus of activity and activity in its immediate surround with the focus inhibited. In terms of human language, the difference will be between linguistic denotation and paralinguistic connotation – between explicit relationships between objects and events as specified through language, on the one hand, and classes of similar relationships, on the other hand. Moreover, insofar as parallel associational fibers connect various cortical regions, this mechanism of 'cognitive generalization' will not be unique to cortical regions joined by the corpus callosum; it will be an ongoing process wherever inhibitory fibers join two regions with corticocortical connecting fibers and which are simultaneously aroused by subcortical mechanisms.

Due solely to the extensive bilateral connections throughout the brainstem, in general, and the reticular activating system, in particular, it is likely that arousal effects are generally bilateral in nature, whereas simultaneous arousal of two intrahemispheric regions would be possible but less inevitable. For this reason, the mirror-image negative mechanism of corticocortical communication would be an incessant and inevitable aspect of *inter*hemispheric communications, whereas it would be less frequent *intra*hemispherically.

In contrast to previous inhibitory models, the mirror-image negative relationship between the cerebral hemispheres implied by the topographical inhibitory model suggests that a unilateral engram would 'switch off' only its own precise mirror-image contralaterally. Column-by-column homotopic inhibition implies a complementary pattern which, although doubly transformed into a mirror-image negative and inevitably somewhat 'faded,' nonetheless contains topographical neural information which is *complementary* to that of the other hemisphere. In other words, whichever hemisphere is not dominant for language (due presumably to anatomical or biochemical asymmetries) will contain complementary contextual information which, although not amenable to precise and coherent expression, is the product of cognitive processing at a level comparable to that of language itself.

5
MAJOR THEMES OF CEREBRAL LATERALITY

The previous chapter might be summarized briefly as an argument for considering the most fundamental functional dichotomy of the cerebral hemispheres of man to be 'language/context.' Yet particularly insofar as some structural and functional asymmetries are also found in other species, it seems likely that the *origins* of cerebral laterality antedate human language functions and consequently that there may be more primal dichotomies than 'language/context.'

Among the more interesting dichotomies previously suggested are those based upon differential hand usage (skilled motor activity versus holding and stabilizing 'contextual' motor skills – Bruner, 1967), emotionality ('approach' and the positive emotions versus 'escape' and the negative emotions – Flor-Henry, 1983), territoriality (movement of self versus map of behavioral territory – Corballis and Morgan, 1978) or concept of 'self' (personal desires and motivations versus those expressed within the group – Jaynes, 1976). Such antecedent dichotomies are of genuine historical interest within the context of the evolution of cerebral asymmetry, but it is not necessarily the case that the evolutionarily early origins of laterality have maintained their central importance throughout evolution and the emergence of modern man. To the contrary, even if lateral specialization arose from the directional twisting of the DNA helix or even prehistoric man's habit of whistling around the campfire, the subsequent use of asymmetric (and, more likely, complementary) brain functions in the realms of language and handedness would undoubtedly have had greater survival value and have slowly become the dominant brain asymmetry.

Judging solely from the clinical significance of the aphasias, it can be said that, even if the language–context dichotomy in man is not evolutionarily primordial, it could well be the *dominant* dichotomy in the modern brain. Moreover if we have correctly identified a callosal mechanism which contributes to the functional dichotomy, then the language–context dichotomy in man suggests a more general dichotomy of neuronal activity which should apply to non-language functions in man and perhaps in other species. That is regardless of the psychological content of the hemispheric activity, any animal with inhibitory forebrain commissures would develop a focus of neuronal activity (particularly as related to skilled motor tasks) and simultaneously a complementary pattern of activity in the contralateral hemisphere. In this

147

more general form the 'focus–context' dichotomy may be broad enough to encompass other dichotomies of cerebral hemisphere function.

It does not follow that all differences between the cerebral hemispheres in man and other species are necessarily the direct result of a focus–context dichotomy, but the pervasiveness of language-related activities in human life suggests that any functional mechanism due to hemispheric relations during language might be predominant and have direct or indirect influences on other forms of hemispheric specialization. The fact that the entire field of hemisphere research originated in clinical examples of asymmetric language capacities may not prove the preeminence of language, but the ability to make sense of the language-related findings must inevitably be a primary concern. In the previous chapter some of the most important issues concerned with the right hemisphere's contribution to language activities have been discussed, but it now remains to review briefly the other areas of known lateral specialization.

Language

The nature of hemispheric specialization has been intensely researched over the past twenty years in both normal and abnormal, human and animal populations. The strength of the conclusions concerning hemispheric differences varies widely depending upon the tasks involved and the subpopulation under study, and debate continues whether or not any single dichotomy can effectively incorporate most or all of the relevant findings. If there is anything approaching consensus, it appears to lie in the general feeling that a neat and clean, single dichotomy will never capture all that the cerebral hemispheres have to offer, and yet that such dichotomies have proven useful in classifying research findings and stimulating further investigations. Still virtually all attempts at characterizing the human cerebral hemispheres in terms of a fundamental dichotomy are based upon the fact that the left hemisphere is superior at language tasks – particularly those requiring speech.

So, let us briefly examine the kinds of evidence from normal subjects that have led to the characterization of the left hemisphere as the 'language hemisphere.' The most basic finding has been that words presented either to the right visual field or the right ear (that is predominantly to the left hemisphere) are recognized more quickly and more accurately than those presented to the right hemisphere (figure 5.1). This asymmetry for language processing has been reported many times and appears to hold true regardless of whether or not the words are nonsense syllables or real words. Because of some effects of eye-scanning, there are some complications with regard to Yiddish, which reads from right to left, and some interesting variations with regard to the ideographic writing systems in the Orient (see pp. 154–6), but generally the asymmetry is found regardless of the language or culture in

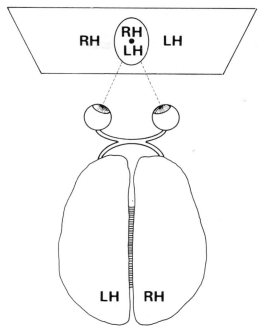

Figure 5.1 Visual laterality effects. Stimuli presented to the center of the visual field will be recorded in both cerebral hemispheres, but those presented several degrees to the right or left of the fixation point will arrive initially in only the left or right hemisphere. The dominant hemisphere for language will be able to read accurately a larger number of words or letters flashed to the contralateral visual field.

about 70–90 percent of the normal subjects in a typical experiment. The effects are stronger in men than in women and more frequently found in right-handers than left-handers, but weaker or reversed in many subjects with psychiatric problems.

In the auditory modality, dichotic listening experiments circumvent the problem of the bilateral coursing of auditory nerve fibers by presenting competing sounds to both ears (figure 5.2). Because of the relatively stronger cortical representation of sounds from the contralateral ear, subjects will normally become cognizant of only one of the stimuli, depending presumably upon the hemisphere which is dominant for such processing. As with visual presentation, the dichotic listening effects are much stronger in the split-brain patients in which the language capacities of the left hemisphere have been isolated from those on the right, but the similarity of results between normal and split-brain subjects offers strong support for considering the left hemisphere to be vastly superior at linguistic processing.

It is of interest, however, that the idea of a uniquely left hemispheric 'speech decoder' is no longer favored (e.g. Bradshaw and Nettleton, 1983). While left-hemispheric superiority in many linguistic – particu-

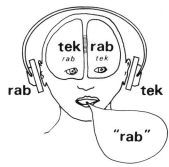

Figure 5.2 Auditory laterality effects. The laterality of auditory processing is less absolute than that of visual processing, so that the dichotic listening technique is usually employed – in which competing sounds are sent to the two ears. Unless attention is deliberately focused toward one ear or the other, normally only one of the words or nonsense syllables will be heard. The 'dominant' hemisphere for phonetic decoding will provide most of the answers.

larly speech – functions is apparent, attempts to define the specific elements of language which are responsible for left-sided advantages have not met with success. This has led to the belief that perhaps the left hemisphere's main superiority is involved in speech *encoding*, and this output capability has some reinforcing effect on speech *decoding*.

At any rate, the superiority of the left hemisphere in dealing with most linguistic tasks, whether in the auditory or visual modality, cannot be doubted. From a review of visual split-field studies, Beaumont (1982) has concluded:

> Words, letters, digits, letter strings and nonsense words are all generally associated with a right visual field [left hemisphere] advantage. Semantic and linguistic parameters have not been clearly shown to be related to this effect. The effect is found with horizontal or vertical presentation.

Superiority of the left hemisphere is not in fact found for *all* language tasks, but those which are commonly studied are so much greater than the asymmetries found in various non-linguistic tasks that a verbal/non-verbal characterization is still the single most accurate dichotomy as related to hemisphere function. It must be emphasized that there are some non-linguistic tasks at which the left hemisphere is superior and some linguistic tasks for which the right hemisphere is also needed, so the 'verbal/non-verbal' dichotomy is not in fact the whole story. Still, it is a large part of it.

Visuospatial functions

Right-hemisphere damage has long been known to lead to a high incidence of visuospatial problems and deficits in moving around in unfamiliar places – with or without the aid of a map. Subsequent testing of the split-brain patients gave further evidence of significant right-hemisphere contributions in deciphering two- and three-dimensional space and in undertaking spatial transformations using the hands (Gazzaniga, 1970). For example, when the split-brain patient's left hand (right hemisphere) is made to draw a three-dimensional object or copy a figure, the fundamental spatial relations among the elements in the drawing are normally found – even if the drawing made by the right-handed individual's untrained left hand appears a bit wobbly. When the left hemisphere (right hand) attempts the same drawing, however, its motor control over the right hand is certain, but the drawing itself contains more stick-figure representations and often shows a loss of perspective and an understanding of three-dimensional geometry.

Nebes (1974) has found that the performance of split-brain subjects differs when the left or right hemisphere is required to perceive the relationship between parts and wholes in performing spatial transformations of visual information. For example, judging which of several circles corresponds to a small arc of a circle is more accurately performed by the right hemisphere than the left. This has led him to suggest that the right hemisphere is, in general, responsible for producing both spatial and 'cognitive' maps of the environment on the basis of incomplete sensory information. Zaidel and Sperry (1974), on the other hand, argue that the left hemisphere uses an analytic strategy in the recognition of faces and complex shapes, whereas the right hemisphere apprehends complex shapes as a unitary Gestalt. Gazzaniga (1970) has emphasized the specifically *manipulo*spatial superiorities of the right hemisphere in the split-brain patients, but again it is the right hemisphere which appears to be more competent in performing spatial transformations.

Evidence for a right hemisphere superiority in the recognition of human faces is also quite strong (e.g. Ley and Bryden, 1979), but the exact nature of the superiority is less certain. That is it may be due to a visuospatial talent of the right hemisphere, the ability to process holistic or Gestalt images, or perhaps the ability to interpret emotions – a significant part of which might be face and trait recognition.

Demonstration of visuospatial superiorities of the right hemisphere in normal subjects has in fact proven more difficult – presumably because of the equalizing effect of the massive commissural communications. To date, there is still no simple tachistoscopic test which produces indisputably left visual field (right hemispheric) advantages of visuospatial tasks which are as distinct as those found for the left hemisphere using the nonsense syllables test. This is perhaps not surprising insofar as – whatever the right hemisphere's unique or relative talents – it *normally* expresses itself *through* the left hemisphere. Still the lack of a simple recognition test superiority by the right hemisphere must be considered a major theoretical problem for the advocates of a fundamental verbal/visuospatial dichotomy for the cerebral hemispheres.

Davidoff (1982) concludes a review of visual split-field studies by noting that:

> Non-verbal tasks have been found to be better performed in the left visual field [right hemisphere] for a variety of what could be called 'lower level', and certainly not categorical, judgments. Such tasks include detection, brightness estimation, color, motion and depth perception, localization, orientation and form discrimination. Of these only a few could be said to give reliable visual field advantages, but if a visual field advantage is obtained it is usually to the left.

The relative weakness of right-hemisphere superiorities at various visuospatial tasks suggests that the unilaterality of the relevant cognitive functions is not as essential nor as absolute as that involved in language. Indeed, it has often been argued that some hemispheric specializations are found on the right simply as a matter of default. That is since the left hemisphere in man has become occupied with important language skills, the 'left over' cortical space on the right (homologous to Broca's and Wernicke's areas) may be 'freed' to do other kinds of processing. This view is not, however, universally accepted. Corballis and Morgan (1978), for example, argue to the contrary that a right-hemispheric visuospatial capability related to territoriality is the likely antecedent specialization – with subsequent left-hemispheric skills filling the 'free space' on the left.

An important variation on the visuospatial theme of right-hemisphere talents is the view that the essential specialization of the right is in the realm of *manipulo*spatial processing. This view is advocated by Gazzaniga and LeDoux (1978), who argue strongly that there is little evidence for fundamentally different modes of *information processing* in the two hemispheres. They maintain that hemispheric differences are more accurately seen as the result of differences in the mechanisms of *utilizing* information. Furthermore, 'most if not all measurable instances of lateralized processing are . . . really by-products of the lateralization of linguistic mechanisms' (p. 63). The neural space homologous to language centers on the left is involved, in their view, in the manipulation of the external world (as well illustrated by a brain-damaged patient in figure 4.2). There are some oddities in this view – notably that the most important neural substrate for manipulospatiality is in posterior (associative or sensory) cortex rather than in anterior (motor) cortex. There is also no obvious 'complementarity' between language, on the one hand, and manipulospatiality, on the other, and in fact they argue that such talents are less evident on the left simply due to the crowding out of such processes in deference to the more important language processes on the left. Finally the abundance of callosal fibers precisely at these regions seems anomalous.

At any rate, it cannot be disputed that both the language functions on the left and the spatial functions on the right are more pronounced when the involvement of the motor apparatus is also required.

Musical functions

Unilateral brain damage can result in the inability to talk, but a preserved ability to sing – or vice versa. The striking capability of some totally aphasic patients to sing a familiar melody – complete with the correct pronunciation and articulation of the lyrics – strongly indicates that the left hemisphere is *not* the only capable controller of the articulatory apparatus. Superior it may be in speech, but the right hemisphere of such patients is capable of similar motor manipulations, provided that it has the aid of a musical melody.

These musical talents of the right hemisphere have led to the suggestion that a fundamental hemispheric dichotomy, at least in man, may be speech on the left side and the prosody of speech (one aspect of which may be the generation of melodies) on the right. Examination of hemispheric differences in normal and split-brain subjects, however, has shown that not all musical talents are resident in the right. Although the right hemisphere is normally superior at recognition of musical chords and melodies (Gordon, 1974), the left hemisphere is now thought to be fundamentally important in the perception of temporal order, tone duration, simultaneity and rhythm (Gordon, 1974) – all of which are important for the recognition or generation of musical melodies.

Musical training and listening strategies have been found to play a role in determining hemispheric contributions to musical perception but, in general, the right hemisphere contributes relatively more to the recognition of chords and the recognition and production of melodies, while the left hemisphere appears to be relatively important in the recognition and production of rhythmic sequences. These hemispheric differences certainly cannot be used in support of a verbal/nonverbal dichotomy, and appear to support a serial processing versus parallel processing characterization. Although it has previously been pointed out that the right hemisphere's superiority at the recognition of melodies, which are clearly serial phenomena, argues against a 'parallel-processing' view of the right hemisphere, it is nonetheless true that many three- and four-note segments of simple melodies add up to recognizable chords. As such, the melody-related talents of the right may not be inconsistent with a parallel 'pattern-recognition' mode of cognition.

The Japanese language

In contrast to the alphabet of English, the Japanese system of writing includes two phonetic systems: the kana (hiragana and katakana) and a domesticated version of the Chinese characters (the kanji). Of particular interest is the fact that, while the kana function in ways similar to the English alphabet, each kanji simultaneously has a very few phonetic readings (usually two) but a definite and circumscribed meaning (usually one, infrequently two). What this unusual dual-writing system (which is unique to Japanese) implies is that the individual elements in the kana writing system have no semantic content until they are collected into a sufficiently long string (similar to words built from the English alphabet). In contrast, although the kanji are phonetically a bit more ambiguous, they are semantically well-defined – whether standing alone or imbedded in a string of kanji and/or kana. For example, although a single phonetic symbol, such as 'テ' (one of the katakana, pronounced 'teh'), has no intrinsic meaning, the single kanji, '手' (which can also be pronounced 'teh' or, alternatively, 'shu'), does have a definite meaning. Whereas the phonetic symbol 'テ' will occur in the present perfect and past perfect of all verbs and is used in countless nouns, adjectives, adverbs, etc., '手' will denote or connote 'hand,' 'arm,' 'manipulation,' 'procedure' or 'reach' in virtually all of its many uses, regardless of the part of speech and regardless of which pronunciation is used. In other words, the kanji symbol '手' (unlike the phonetic symbol 'テ') has a definite (if broad) meaning and consequently a definite context and place within a semantic network whenever it is read.

Since the writing of both the kana and the kanji symbols is done by the right hand (left hemisphere), it would not be surprising if the left hemisphere were superior at the recognition and manipulation of both, but the difference between them in terms of inherent semantic content should produce measurable differences. Whereas the kana are merely the phonetic tools used by the left hemisphere for constructing words and sentences (which have semantic content only as a sequence of symbols), the kanji are themselves semantic units. Whereas the kana are symbols which correspond to defined movements and positions of the organs of speech, the kanji characteristically correspond to one or several phonemes in succession, but they have meaning. The kanji alone are therefore imbedded in a complex, but finite and often well-defined system of semantic associations.

The significance of this unique dual-writing system is that the kanji should be less confined to the left hemisphere temporal lobe regions specialized for phonetic encoding/decoding and more involved in the semantic systems in, presumably, association cortex in both cerebral hemispheres.

Empirically it has been shown that in normal subjects there are laterality effects in the processing of kana and kanji and that kanji tend to have more bilateral representation (e.g. Sasanuma *et al.*, 1980; Hatta, 1981). In general the normal left hemisphere advantage for linguistic processing found for the kana disappears or is reversed when kanji are used as the test stimuli. Perhaps the clearest indication of right-hemispheric involvement in kanji processing was found by Hatta (1981) in a Stroop test. He presented words written in either kanji or kana to the left or right visual field. The usual Stroop technique was used in which words meaning green, yellow, red or blue were presented in an appropriate or inappropriate color. The task for the subject was simply to read the word, trying to ignore the actual color of the presentation. Measuring the time until the response, Hatta found no difference due to visual field for the kana words, but a significant (50 percent) increase in time required to respond when the kanji words were presented to the left visual field (right hemisphere) than to the right visual field. In accordance with the usual interpretation of Stroop tests, this finding was thought to indicate greater 'interference' of the color in the right hemisphere on the reading of the character – i.e. a greater involvement of the right hemisphere in reading the kanji than in reading the kana.

The situation is not, however, as simple as a kana-left versus kanji-right dichotomy. The principal complicating factor has been the finding that right hemisphere *damage* rarely affects the reading of kanji characters. Although there have been some striking examples of individuals with callosal damage and subsequent deficits in kanji but not kana reading (Sugishita *et al.*, 1978), the great majority of patients studied thus far have shown deficits in kana or kanji reading only after left-hemisphere damage (Iwata *et al.*, 1982). The fact that deficits in reading kana and kanji can be dissociated following circumscribed brain damage is of considerable neuropsychological interest because the dissociation indicates different intracortical processing routes for the two kinds of writing system. It is, however, an unresolved issue why a relatively strong laterality effect can be obtained in normal subjects, while the bulk of evidence from brain-damaged patients does not support the idea of significant right hemispheric involvement in kanji reading.

As evident from the above, although the empirical issue remains uncertain, it is worth noting that a 'language/context' dichotomy suggests an interesting hemispheric asymmetry in the Japanese language. Since each kana has no intrinsic meaning and inevitably occurs in hundreds and thousands of different contexts of differing semantic content, there is no obvious prediction concerning hemisphere differences when identifying the 'context' of an isolated phoneme – simply because there is no inherent 'context.' In both English and Japanese, although a left hemisphere superiority is expected for phoneme or letter identification (recognition, recall, etc.), what, for example in English, is the context within which 'h's are found? Is there any connotative implication of all 'r's or is there any conceptual constant in the 'str' complex? Probably not, and negative answers are equally certain for the Japanese kana. That is insofar as the phonetic systems in language are inherently linked to the proper control of the motor organs involved in speech, the left-hemispheric phoneme encoder has no obvious right-hemisphere counterpart: there is no 'context' to an isolated, arbitrary phoneme. In Japanese, however, the network of associations for each individual kanji is finite and each exists within a well-developed 'semantic network.' Although the origins of the kanji may be as arbitrary and inherently meaningless as the symbols in any written language, each of the many hundreds of kanji comes to be used within a restricted semantic framework and is eventually understood as having a single amorphous meaning.

A similar situation is found in the Latin and Greek stems and root words found throughout the English lexicon. Because most such root words cannot stand alone and have undergone many large and small changes which often obscure their origins, root words in English do not maintain as autonomous an existence as the kanji. Nonetheless the idea that a kanji could maintain a 'single, rather amorphous meaning' is easily understood by considering the meanings of, for example, the Latin root words 'com' (with, together, in association with, etc.) and 'plex' (plaited, plied, intermingled, etc.). As in the case of English words built from several root words, knowing the meaning of the individual kanji does not necessarily produce the precise meaning of the compound word, but a rough indication of same can usually be obtained. Moreover the diversity of words within which the Latin roots are used is such that a single *precise* meaning for each stem is not possible, but a somewhat vague meaning is apparent from the sum total of usages in English. In the Japanese language the stand alone meaning of each kanji character is clearer than the meaning of Latin roots for two main reasons: (i) the kanji do not undergo morphological changes depending upon usage (or neighboring letters within a word); and (ii) the kanji must be studied for the Japanese individual to become literature, whereas knowledge of Latin and Greek may enhance English literacy, but is not essential.

For this reason, it is expected that, unlike the phonetic symbols, the ideographic characters will elicit more in the way of contextual meaning and associations in the right hemisphere than the intrinsically meaningless phonetic units, the kana. It is therefore likely that semantic paralexias would be more easily generated with kanji than with kana and more easily in the right hemisphere than in the left. Such a test remains to be done.

Can other hemispheric dichotomies be related to 'focus–context'?

If the 1960s were an era of renewed interest in hemispheric differences and the 1970s an era of proposals concerning 'fundamental' dichotomies, the 1980s have been one long, cold shower. No single dichotomy has been shown to encompass all experimental findings and some dichotomies seem to relate consistently to but few, if any, empirical data. Realizing that there is a pervasive pessimism surrounding all discussions of neat hemispheric dichotomies, I have nonetheless suggested still another dichotomy based originally upon the growing realization of important right-hemispheric contributions to high-level, particularly linguistic, cognition. Certainly as one more 'partial truth,' the language–context dichotomy has some validity, and has been developed in slightly different ways by various neuropsychologists – notably Kinsbourne, Gardner and Geschwind. It must be said, however, that in its more generalized form of 'a focus of unilaterally generated cortical activity versus a contextual mirror-image negative,' the focus–context dichotomy should theoretically manifest itself in various other areas of psychological reseach where hemispheric specialization is known to come into play.

To be sure, if the language–context dichotomy had been developed in the previous chapters *without* reference to a causal callosal mechanism, then it could simply be argued that the language–context dichotomy is one example of a high-level cognitive dichotomy – possibly functioning alongside or resulting from other high- and low-level hemispheric dichotomies. Alone, advocacy of a characterization of the cerebral hemispheres which emphasizes high-level hemispheric *complementarity* is, I believe, a worthwhile mission, but implication of a neural mechanism demands that the suggested dichotomy has broad generality.

In fact generalization of the proposed callosal mechanism to other species remains somewhat problematical because of species differences in callosal termination, etc., but if a topographical inhibitory role for the corpus callosum (between regions of association cortex) is to be postulated for language functions, then similar effects certainly must be obtainable for various *non-language* functions in human beings. At this point, only some rather general remarks can be made, but it seems likely that the fate of this hypothesis concerning the role of the corpus callosum may be decided by the ability or inability of callosal inhibition to account for both contextual and non-language (visuospatial, musical, etc.) aspects of hemispheric specialization.

The 'serial/parallel' characterization of the cerebral hemispheres is one previously suggested dichotomy which implies hemispheric differences not unlike those of the focus–context dichotomy. The latter, however, may provide some theoretical advantages over the former, primarily in that the inhibitory callosal hypothesis does *not* require postulation of unknown intrahemispheric neuronal mechanisms which result in the serial/parallel differences in information processing.

In analogy with computer systems, the serial/parallel dichotomy suggests that the left hemisphere is a sequential 'processor,' whose primary responsibility is the 'linearization' of skilled motor acts, particularly language – choosing the proper sequence of articulatory movements to build phonemes, phonemes to build words and words to build sentences. The right hemisphere, in this view, is somehow capable of simultaneous or parallel processing of many such smaller elements to build Gestalts at various semantic levels. Specialization for temporal sequencing, rhythm and goal-directed movements, on the one hand, and spatial, holistic patterning, on the other, then appear to be natural consequences of these asymmetrically located processors, but the underlying mechanism remains unexplained.

The focus–context dichotomy may provide a mechanism in the following way. That is the left hemisphere might be employed in the task of 'linearizing' language tasks (etc.) while, as a consequence of callosal inhibition, each instant of neuronal processing on the left would generate a more diffuse neuronal engram on the right. There is therefore no need to maintain that the right-sided neuronal hardware differs significantly from that on the left. On the contrary a 'parallel-processing' mode would be a direct consequence of the inhibition by the focal cortical pattern on the left, of its right-sided homolog and a consequent excitation of 'other,' peripherally located regions of cortex. The 'parallelism' of the right hemisphere would then not be due, in the first instance, to anatomical features of right-hemisphere hardware, but rather would be due to functional, physiological processes which are asymmetric solely as a consequence of unilateral 'dominance' for a given motor task. The inhibitory mechanism may thereby avoid the need to speculate about fundamental cellular asymmetries of an unknown kind (which are presumed to lead to left-hemispheric sequential processing and right-hemispheric parallel processing). In other words, asymmetries of information processing may simply be a consequence of topographical inhibition and the resultant, transient 'mirror-image negative' pattern of cortical activity.

Conclusions

A final word about hemispheric dichotomies is yet needed. Contrary to many current suggestions of 'separate personalities' embodied in the two hemispheres, the two halves of the brain are structurally and functionally far more similar than dissimilar. Granted that the split-brain patients display some interesting (if quite abnormal) antagonisms between the 'two brains' and acknowledging that many serious people have spent countless hours working on techniques to emulate the split-brain condition in normal subjects, still the fact remains that brains are 'integrated' via the forebrain commissures and present to the conscious self a unified view of the world. The differences between the hemispheres and the validity of psychological dichotomies must be viewed within the context of an organ whose primary function appears to provide its owner with an 'integrated mind.'

6

RELEVANT ANIMAL EXPERIMENTS

Since the publication of Kuhn's book, *The Structure of Scientific Revolutions* (1970), many scientists have come to think of scientific research in terms of 'paradigms' and their eventual overthrow in light of 'crisis' facts. Particularly for the experimentalist, this view of science is attractive, insofar as it suggests that careful experimental methodology together with an eye for detecting unusual and potentially critical anomalies is the key to scientific progress.

Historically this approach has been one way in which progress has been made, but I am not convinced that – except in retrospect – crisis facts will often stand out clearly enough to fire revolutions without a clear-cut theoretical alternative within which the new data can fit. To be sure, anomalies may be more obvious in disciplines which have a fundamental mathematical basis but, particularly in psychology, I believe it is fair to say that anomalous experimental results are not all that unusual. Revolutions do not occur with similar frequency simply because the overwhelming emphasis in the 'young' (central dogma-less) science of psychology is on methodological rigor and statistical precision, rather than on theoretical coherence. There is good historical reason for this insistence on a hard-headed scientific psychology, but it nevertheless seems odd that a topic as broad and complex as brain science should be a predominantly empirical endeavor, while departments of theoretical biology, theoretical chemistry and theoretical physics are recognized as valid and worthwhile disciplines which complement and contribute to the related experimental disciplines.

I would not argue for a return to introspectionist psychology, but it is important to recognize the theoretical underpinnings of all scientific research – simply as a means for evaluating anomalous empirical findings. Undoubtedly many anomalies are anomalous for uninteresting and trivial reasons, but some findings cannot be easily explained away and clearly point in unexpected directions. Perhaps the most embarrassing fact which does not fit neatly into modern neuroscience (but has not been elevated to the status of 'crisis finding') is the extremely normal psychological functioning of people with hydrocephalus. The embarrassment of such cases is that they are psychologically normal or only slightly subnormal, and yet have only a small percentage of the brain matter – specifically neocortical white and grey matter – which most people have. Due to faulty drainage of cerebrospinal fluid, much of the intracranial space has been used up solely for holding the watery liquor within the cerebral ventricles, and in some cases nearly 95 percent of the cerebral hemispheres is not brain, but water.

Although I can offer no explanation for their normality, I suggest that such empirical facts do not constitute a crisis for brain science simply because there is no viable alternative to the neuron theory of brain function. We are therefore forced to waffle and wave our hands saying that in some cases very little brain matter is needed, while contrarily insisting that the normally massive brain is the essential substrate of the human mind and the instrument which distinguishes us among the animal kingdom!

The example of hydrocephalus is a good one, not because there is much potential in a cerebrospinal fluid theory of mind, but because it points out that – rightly or wrongly – we are all rather heavily dependent upon certain fundamental assumptions which, in all honesty, we do not often think about. Those tacit assumptions about the mind and brain are sometimes called 'philosophy' and sometimes 'theory,' but always held tenaciously – often in the face of potentially 'critical,' paradigm-altering data. In our minds, such anomalies, exceptions and embarrassing facts are neatly filed away under 'areas for future research,' 'dubious findings because of possible methodological problems' or simply 'suspect investigator.'

Sometimes we may be right in stubbornly refusing to face up to the reported anomalies and UFOs of brain science but, amidst the rather large collection of findings which lie outside of current theories of brain function, it is likely that there are a few dozen genuine 'crisis' facts which, someday with hindsight, historians will note as the early, unnoticed precursors of the (eventual) revolution in our understanding of the brain.

Without a central dogma or predominant paradigm, psychology cannot be expected to undergo a Kuhnian 'revolution,' but there are several sets of experimental data which I believe deserve wider appreciation. Those and related issues will be reviewed in this chapter.

Association cortex and the intrahemispheric convergence of sensory pathways

The primary sensory maps on the neocortex (reviewed in chapter 2) are the first means for representing information at the cortical level, but their subsequent manipulation and association is still required to allow for polymodal and supramodal information processing. The neuronal physiology of how such manipulations could occur is not well understood, but some questions concerning where the information from different sensory modalities is brought together have been answered in anatomical studies. One such study by Jones and Powell (1970) is a modern classic of this kind.

The study was done using rhesus monkeys and is therefore thought to provide solid indications of how the human brain is also organized. The strategy was to make lesions at areas of the cortex which are known to be major recipients of primary sensory afferents, and then to study the pattern of axonal degeneration which other areas suffer as a consequence. Those areas which showed degeneration were then lesioned in other animals, and their connections then studied, and so on. Each of the major sensory modalities (vision, audition and somesthesis) were studied separately and each stage of processing within each modality was also studied separately – resulting in the sacrifice of a total of twenty-three animals. In this way the anatomy of individual steps in the processing of sensory information could be identified, and the results gathered together to provide a picture of the entire sequential processing that presumably occurs in any normal brain.

The results are presented in table 6.1 and figure 6.1 and they are generalized to the human brain in figure 6.2.

A remarkable aspect of these results is that distinct regions of unimodal and polymodal processing regions were found at virtually every major area of the entire neocortex. Strictly speaking some uncertainty remains with regard to the nature of the sensory processing in the angular and supramarginal gyri of the human brain since these areas are not developed in the monkey brain. However, insofar as those gyri are thought to be expansions of the monkey's superior temporal sulcus (Jones and Powell, 1970), it can be concluded that the *first* cortical region of polysensory information processing is in the inferior

Table 6.1 The cascade of sensory information in the cortex

Source: Jones and Powell (1970).

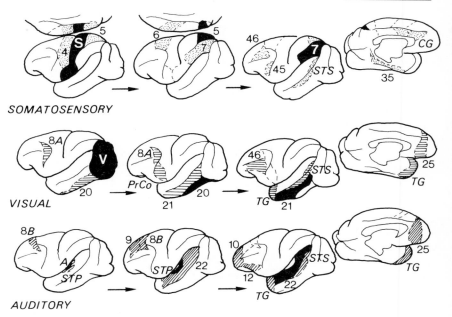

SOMATOSENSORY

VISUAL

AUDITORY

Figure 6.1 The convergence of sensory pathways in the rhesus monkey (after Jones and Powell, 1970). In each brain diagram, the blackened region indicates where cortical lesions were made; the stipling or shading indicates regions where axonal degeneration was later found. Abbreviations are as follows: A, primary auditory cortex; CG, cingulate cortex; PrCo, precentral agranular field; S, primary somatosensory cortex; STP, superior temporal plane; STS, superior temporal sulcus; TG, area TG; V, primary visual cortex. Numbers refer to Brodmann's areas.

parietal lobe (approximately the region known as Wernicke's area). The limited and yet controversial capacity for monkeys to generalize from one sensory modality to another may be a consequence of the limited development of this part of the brain. Subsequent to polymodal association at this region of the parietal lobe, it can be seen in figure 6.2 that much of the limbic cortex receives polymodal input and is effectively a form of association cortex.

Given these routes over which information in different modalities is brought together, it is of interest to calculate the number of ways in which sensory information might be permutated. Limiting ourselves to only touch, vision and hearing, and given the possibility of both topographical excitation and inhibition, as well as mirror-image reversals (see pp. 163–75), already a tremendous number of permutations of sensory information is possible. A few such possibilities are illustrated in figure 6.3. The actual patterns shown in this figure should not be taken too seriously, but it is abundantly clear that – before slipping into despair or speculation about unknown mechanisms of 'supramodal' information processing – we should explore the significance of the

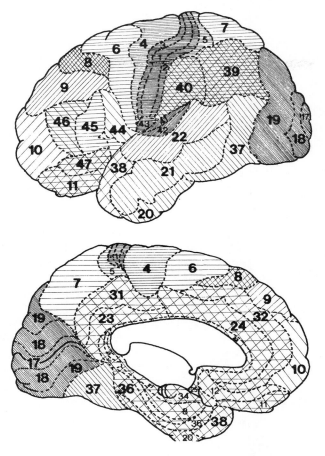

Figure 6.2 Sensory convergence in the human brain. Generalization of the findings in the rhesus monkey to the human cortex suggests that most of the cortex is involved in 'unimodal' sensory processing, but important portions of the parietal, temporal and limbic lobes are 'bimodal' or 'trimodal'. The first region of trimodal association is at parietal cortex, areas 39 and 40.

permutations made possible by the known mechanisms of intracortical communications. Clearly a considerable variety of 'maps' can be produced in response to the input of three essentially static sensory images along the major input channels. If indeed topographical inhibition is a mechanism for generalization, does the brain really require 'abstract' information-processing modes?

Mirror-image transfers across the forebrain commissures

Since the cerebral hemispheres are connected predominantly by means of homotopic fibers, theoretically a pattern of activity in one hemi-

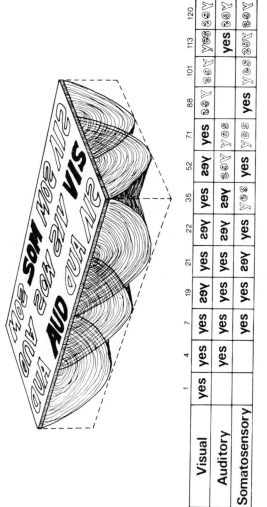

	1	4	7	19	21	22	35	52	71	88	101	113	120
Visual	yes	yes		yes	yes	yes	yes	yes	yes	yes	yes	yes	yes
Auditory		yes	yes	yes	yes	yes	yes	yes	yes			yes	yes
Somatosensory			yes	yes	yes	yes	yes	yes	yes	yes	yes	yes	yes

Figure 6.3 The permutations of sensory information. If excitatory and inhibitory topographical mapping of visual, auditory and somesthetic information occurs, then three items of information can be permuted 720 (6!) times.

sphere could be transferred to the contralateral hemisphere over those fibers as an exact (although probably 'faded' or degraded) 'mirror-image.' The fact that children and animals commonly have considerable difficulty in distinguishing between horizontal mirror-image letters (b and d, p and q) but have less difficulty distinguishing between vertical mirror-images (u and n, p and b) suggests that there is something special about the left–right pairs. Starting with the observations of Orton (1937) on the reading disabilities of children, psychologists have often speculated about a possible relationship between these left–right confusions and the left–right symmetry of the brain. The nature of the neural mechanisms involved remains a controversial subject, but it is well known that mirror-image movements of the hands are common in babies, tend to disappear with age in normal children, but persist in various pathological states (Abercrombie *et al.*, 1964). Further discussion of this topic can be found in *The Psychology of Left and Right* by Corballis and Beale (1976) and in Critchley's monograph entitled *Mirror Writing* (1958).

My own introduction to this topic was through my son who, at the age of two, had an interesting tendency to write his name in a normal left-to-right direction with his *right* hand, but in a right-to-left direction – with the letters also reversed – with his *left* hand (figure 6.4). Mirror-image reversals are of course not uncommon among children, but they are usually limited to individual letters or numbers. The reversal of entire words depending upon the hand in use is probably less common, but it can be understood as a complete reversal of all hand and arm movements controlled by the two hemispheres. As will be discussed below, the reversal is probably not a perceptual confusion insofar as both hemispheres are (contrary to Orton's belief) presented with veridical images of the external world. But it is easy to imagine that a cortical memory representation of a motor sequence needed to write a particular shape could be mirror-image reversed in its transferral from one hemisphere (hand) to the other. Mirror-image writing may therefore be the result of the usage of a unilaterally established engram after it has been transmitted (excitatorily?) across the corpus callosum.

As interesting as such anecdotal findings may be, they can never become the basis for a scientific psychology, although they can provide the motivation to investigate possible causal mechanisms. A good, if yet controversial, example of an analytic study is that of Noble (1966, 1968). Reasoning that the homotopicity of callosal fibers could be the mechanism for left–right confusions, he severed the optic chiasma in rhesus monkeys in order that visual stimuli sent to one eye would then be sent directly to only one of the cerebral hemispheres. In this way the mechanisms of commissural transfer could be studied when the other eye was opened and the previously trained eye was closed. The experimental set-up is shown in figure 6.5.

LEFT HAND　　　　**RIGHT HAND**

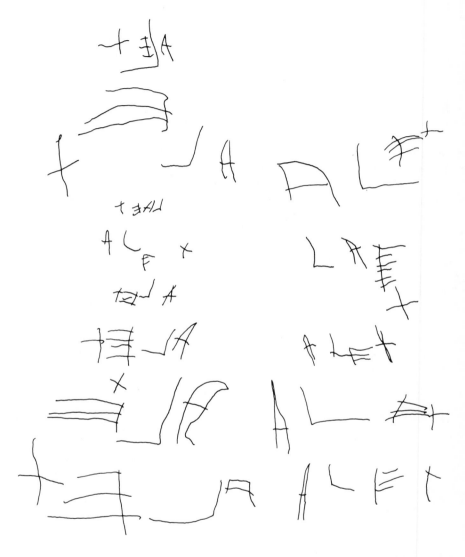

Figure 6.4 Examples of right-to-left writing by a 2-year-old using his right hand and complete left-to-right reversal of words and letters using his left hand. The writing samples were obtained without prompting other than 'Can you write your name?' over a three-week period, after which he became strongly left-handed with normal reading and writing abilities.

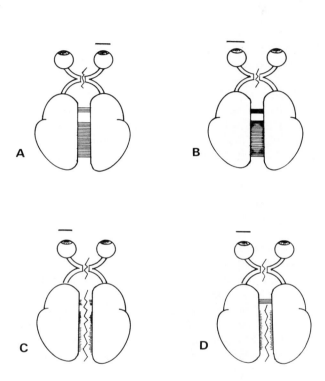

Figure 6.5 The experimental design used by Noble (1968). (A) The monkeys with sectioned optic chiasma were trained to discriminate between horizontal mirror-image stimuli and between vertical mirror-image stimuli to obtain a food reward. One eye was occluded using an opaque contact lens. The monkeys were then tested for the same task, but using the contralateral eye and cerebral hemisphere. The three major test conditions were: corpus callosum and anterior commissure intact (B), both commissures cut (C), and the anterior commissure intact, but the corpus callosum cut (D). The monkeys were more confused by the incorrect horizontal mirror-image stimulus when the anterior commissure was intact (conditions B and D).

The fundamental theoretical prediction was that if the visual stimulus is stored as a topographical map on the cortex, then its interhemispheric transfer would result in its left–right reversal and therefore a preference for the *incorrect* (mirror-image, left–right reversed) stimulus when the contralateral hemisphere was tested. Since a left-to-right reversal does not affect the shape of vertical mirror-image pairs (figure 6.5), a similar incorrect response to vertically symmetrical stimuli was not expected.

Two notable results were obtained – the first discussed by Noble, but since disputed (Butler, 1979) and the second noted by Achim and Corballis (1977). First, as predicted, testing of the untrained hemisphere on the monkeys' choices between the left–right pairs showed a definite preference for the shape which was the mirror-image reversal of the learned (correct) shape. The vertical mirror-image shapes were not confused. Because of changes in the direction of attention with eye, Corballis and Beale (1976) and Butler (1979) have argued that this main effect is likely to be due to a rather uninteresting 'misperception' of the stimuli, rather than mirror-image reversal.

The interpretation of the main finding of commissural reversal thus remains equivocal, but a secondary effect of possibly more significance was noted by Achim and Corballis (1977). That is on examining Noble's data, they found that, regardless of the subsequent status of the corpus callosum (cut or intact), the monkeys which had intact anterior commissures showed much greater confusion concerning the horizontal mirror-image stimuli than those which had undergone section of this tract. Although the two groups with anterior commissure intact or sectioned showed similar speeds of learning the correct shape (348 versus 323 sessions) and made a similar number of errors (141 versus 117) when tested with the *vertical* mirror-images, when they were made to deal with the left–right pairs, the intact group was significantly slower (656 versus 226 sessions) and made significantly more errors (266 versus 94). At the very least, this finding indicates different functions for the anterior commissure and the corpus callosum (see pp. 170–5). It is worth emphasizing that in this experiment the corpus callosum apparently did not produce mirror-image *excitatory* reversal of the shapes, but the anterior commissure did.

Several years after Noble's study, Corballis and Beale (1976, chapter 6, 'Interhemispheric mirror-image reversals') reviewed these and related experiments and have argued that the reversal is unlikely to occur at the level of *perception*, but may be due to commissural reversals of *memory* representations (figure 6.6). Whether or not mirror-image reversals of memory representations could be helpful in generalizing the nature of the perceived objects, as suggested by Corballis and Beale (1976), remains unclear.

Finally mention should be made of the fact that mirror-image movements of the limbs are often seen in certain neurological patients.

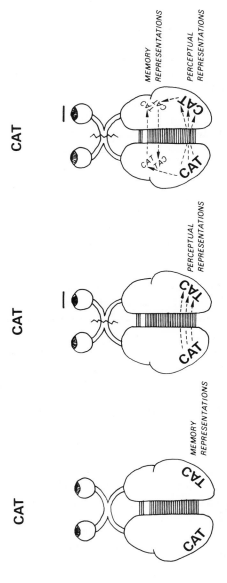

Figure 6.6 Three possible mechanisms of excitatory interhemispheric transfer. In light of the incorrect anatomy of Orton's suggestion (A) and the inconclusiveness of Noble's experiments (B), Corballis and Beale (1976) have suggested a process of mirror-image reversal of 'memory representations' (C) to explain the phenomenon of mirror-image confusions in children. In this view, there is no reversal of 'perceptual representations' at early stages of cortical processing, but high level reversals of 'memory representations' may occur via the corpus callosum.

When a right-handed individual suffers a left-sided stroke, hemiplegia is common and the patient must then learn to write with the unfavored hand. Particularly when hurried or when attention is lax, mirror-image writing frequently occurs (Critchley, 1958). That the mirror-writing is not simply a consequence of abnormal effects of the injured hemisphere acting on the normal right hemisphere is indicated by the fact that similar effects are found in individuals who have suffered damage to the favored hand itself (Schott, 1980). In other words there is a tendency for mirror-writing in *normal* brains which are forced to use the non-preferred hand for skilled movements normally done by the preferred hand. It therefore seems likely that the tendency to make mirror movements is an entirely normal phenomenon – although generally suppressed in the intact adult. Although most speculation about mirror movements has focused on the forebrain commissures, the actual mechanisms remain unknown. Schott (1980) has recently noted:

> There is a long history of the concept of physiological inhibition of bimanual synkinetic movements. . . . This inhibitory mechanism has been considered to develop with maturation, to be deficient in 'idiots' and to be damaged in the presence of certain central nervous system disorders.

The tendency for acallosal patients to show increased mirror movements (Milner, 1983) suggests that the inhibitory mechanism may work via the corpus callosum and to become increasingly strong with the slow maturation of this tract.

The unilateral engram

In a series of studies, Doty and colleagues have examined the mechanisms of callosal transfer of learned responses in monkeys and have advocated the idea that unilateral engram formation may not be unique to man (Doty *et al.* 1973, 1977, 1979). Their conclusions can be summarized in three statements: (i) the corpus callosum enables each hemisphere to have *access* to memory traces stored in the other hemisphere; (ii) it controls the formation of engrams in such a way that, in some situations, an engram is found in only one hemisphere; and (iii) the corpus callosum and anterior commissure are involved in interhemispheric communications in different ways.

The first experiment described below is atypical of callosal studies in finding unilateral engram formation. Others (Butler, 1968; Hamilton, 1977) found bilateral engram formation, but there is an important difference between these experiments. Doty *et al.* used direct stimulation of the visual cortex as their 'external' stimulus, whereas others have used visual stimulation to the retina. The principal difference between these techniques lies in the absence or presence of brainstem effects. When the retina is stimulated, *bilateral* brainstem effects are inevitable;

it is found that the convergence of both 'arousal' effects and cortical information is sufficient to produce bilateral memories. When the cortex itself is directly stimulated, however, the absence of brainstem arousal may be the crucial factor preventing bilateral engram formation. Far from invalidating Doty's experiment, the strictly cortical nature of their stimulus may in fact more closely simulate the cortically generated language of man.

The evidence offered in support of the three conclusions noted above is both of a very general kind and of a more specific kind obtained in animal experiments. The general argument is quite simply that language engrams are found in the left hemisphere in most people: despite massive interhemispheric cross-talk, left-hemispheric damage or left-hemispheric anesthetization will leave the right hemisphere incapable of speech. At the same time, however, normal people do not suffer from the split-brain syndrome: when an object is presented to the left hand, left visual field or left ear, no problems are experienced in sending that information from the right hemisphere to the left hemisphere for an appropriate verbal response. There must consequently be a callosal mechanism which somehow allows 'access' to information in one hemisphere by the other hemisphere, but *without entailing engram duplication*. Doty and Negrao (1973) note:

> Extensive evidence from man conclusively shows that most engrams of language are unilateral. Whether this is the rule or the exception in the formation of engrams is not known. However, the consistent formation of bilateral engrams would halve the mnemonic capacity of the brain and thus seems, *a priori*, an unlikely arrangement.

Two of the more interesting animal experiments reported by Doty *et al.* are as follows. Macaque monkeys can be trained to press a lever to receive a food reward in response to a mild electrical stimulation of the striate cortex (which in human subjects is said to produce an illusory, but painless visual shower of 'phosphenes'). Having trained a normal monkey to respond to such stimulation, it can be tested for its response to stimulation of contralateral (homotopically situated, but untrained) striate cortex. Invariably the monkeys show the same response. When portions of the cortex other than contralateral striate cortex are similarly stimulated, however, no response is elicited (figure 6.7(A), (B)).

The next stage of the experiment involves sectioning selected interhemispheric commissures. If both the anterior commissure and the corpus callosum are cut prior to training, there is no response to stimulation of the striate cortex in the 'untrained' hemisphere. In other words, the information appears to travel over the forebrain commissures, rather than through the brainstem.

Doty and colleagues then asked whether the 'engram' has been laid down bilaterally because of the forebrain commissures, *or* alternatively

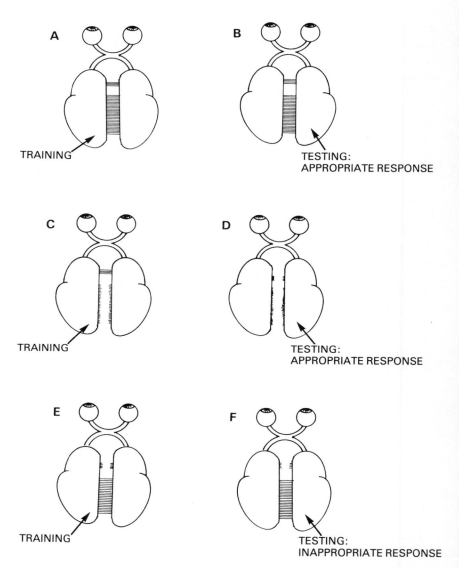

Figure 6.7 The relay of information across the anterior commissure, but not across the corpus callosum, in the Doty *et al.* (1973, 1977, 1979) experiments. In the training sessions the monkeys were trained to respond to mild electrical stimulation at a site on visual cortex (A). When the commissures were intact, the monkeys responded appropriately to contralateral visual cortex stimulation, but not to other contralateral or ipsilateral stimulation (B). When the corpus callosum was sectioned prior to training (C), and the anterior commissure was cut before testing, stimulation of contralateral visual cortex still produced the appropriate response (D). If, however, the anterior commissure was cut prior to training (E), training with or without sectioning of the corpus callosum did *not* result in appropriate responses to contralateral visual cortex stimulation (F).

whether the engram has been somehow 'read out' from the trained hemisphere by the untrained hemisphere. By carrying out experiments in which either the anterior commissure or the corpus callosum was severed prior to training, they have found the following:

(i) If the anterior commissure is kept intact while the corpus callosum is split prior to training, then subsequent to the cutting of the anterior commissure, the monkey responds appropriately to the stimulation of the striate cortex of the 'untrained' hemisphere – as though now both hemispheres independently know the significance of the cortical stimulation (figure 6.7(C), (D)).

Conversely (ii) if the corpsus callosum is kept intact with the anterior commissure severed prior to training, then subsequent cutting of the corpus callosum makes the monkeys incapable of responding appropriately to the stimulation of the untrained hemisphere. In this case, although the callosal fibers were presumably functioning normally during the training of one hemisphere, when the other hemisphere was not allowed callosal access to the information in the trained hemisphere, it was found not to have been trained in tandem with the stimulated hemisphere (figure 6.7(F)). They concluded that: (i) the anterior commissure acts to establish bilateral engrams, whereas (ii) the corpus callosum does not establish bilateral engrams, but allows for 'access' to unilateral engrams.

It is as though the anterior commissure were capable of *excitatory relay* of the engram in one hemisphere over to the other hemisphere – thus allowing bilateral engram formation, whereas the corpus callosum can only 'access' contralateral information, but not duplicate it. This difference between the anterior commissure and the corpus callosum is of interest in the light of Achim and Corballis's (1977) report of the anterior commissure effect in Noble's experiment (1968). Again Noble's monkeys were found to be confused about which of the horizontal mirror-image stimuli was the correct one but, regardless of the condition of the corpus callosum, far more confused if the anterior commissure had been intact during training. In both the Doty and the Noble experiments, therefore, it appears that the anterior commissure had transmitted an image to the other hemisphere – thus producing contradictory images in the two hemispheres. What, therefore, does the corpus callosum do? If, indeed, the anterior commissure works by means of *excitatory* relay, could the corpus callosum be working by means of an *inhibitory* informational relay?

That the corpus callosum is involved in the (excitatory or inhibitory) communication of specific information rather than simply 'arousal' is indicated by a second experiment performed by Doty and colleagues. It is well known from previous studies that when the amygdalae are removed bilaterally from the Macaque monkey, it no longer fears its natural enemy, man. This finding has long been cited as evidence for the amygdala's role in emotional behavior, but Doty *et al.* (1973) have made use of this marked behavioral change to study commissural functions. In their experiment, in addition to cutting the anterior commissure and the anterior portion of the corpus callosum (leaving the posterior portion intact), they cut the optic tract going to one hemisphere and removed the amygdala in the other hemisphere (figure 6.8(A)). They then found that the monkeys still acted with characteristic fear of man and fled to the far side of the cage at his approach. When, however, the posterior corpus callosum was later cut, the 'seeing' hemisphere was no longer capable of sending its fearful signals contralaterally. The monkey's visual behavior remained unchanged, but the significance of the sight of man was lost. Apparently the intact amygdala in one hemisphere had no access to visual information in the other hemisphere.

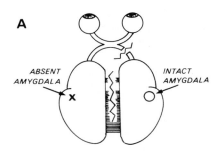

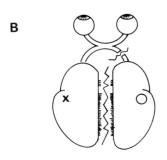

Figure 6.8 The state of the monkey brain in a second experiment by Doty *et al.* (1973, 1977, 1979). (A) The optic tract was cut and the amygdala removed from the only hemisphere which can then directly receive visual information. With the anterior commissure and anterior two-thirds of the corpus callosum also sectioned, monkeys reacted with characteristic fear at the sight of man. (B) Subsequent cutting of the posterior portion of the corpus callosum makes the monkey unafraid of man, suggesting that the relevant visual information no longer reached the intact amygdala.

This experiment poses a major difficulty for the 'alerting' hypothesis of callosal functions (Guiard, 1980) for the following reason. Although the commissural fibers to the amygdala (via the anterior commissure and possibly via the anterior corpus callosum) were severed prior to testing, the significance of the visual information sent to the amygdala-less hemisphere across the posterior corpus callosum was sufficient to make the monkey fearful. Behaviorally, that is, the monkey was appropriately aroused and fearful despite the fact that commissural fibers leading directly to the amygdala were absent. Subsequent to the sectioning of the remaining callosal fibers, however, the monkey was not aroused – a fact which can most easily be explained by a lack of visual information reaching the intact amygdala (rather than a lack of arousal effects coursing to the contralateral amygdala over a tortuous route across the posterior callosum and through blinded visual cortex).

It should be mentioned that Doty and colleagues have suggested that the corpus callosum may normally have inhibitory effects (missing in the callosal agenesis patients), but they have not offered hypotheses concerning the mechanism of callosal 'access' to contralateral engrams. Clearly a diffuse inhibition of contralateral cortex would not serve the required purpose, but if cortical *information* can be transferred by means of topographical inhibition, then a possible mechanism is in sight.

Cerebral dominance in animals

The overwhelming evidence for asymmetry of function of the human cerebral hemispheres has led to two distinct schools of thought concerning possible laterality effects in other species. The first is that hemispheric asymmetry is likely to be a necessary (if not sufficient) condition for the emergence of human language and therefore likely to be as unique to *Homo sapiens* as is symbolic communication. The second school of thought is that, given the fact of biological evolution and the genetic similarities between man and other animal species, it is extremely unlikely that human asymmetries are without precedent in the animal kingdom.

These two perspectives appear at first glance to be mutually exclusive – one viewing hemispheric specialization as an extremely important aspect of the characteristically *human* aspects of brain function and the other seeing human laterality effects (and all other neural phenomena) as part of a biological continuum. A compromise position between these two extremes is, however, worth considering. That is, although not unique to *Homo sapiens*, unilateral engram formation may be an unusually efficient way to store information. It may therefore be correct to emphasize its importance for higher brain functions, but a mistake to believe that only certain of the large primates have discovered its benefits!

Empirically the most clear-cut brain asymmetry in the animal kingdom is the demonstration of distinct left-hemisphere dominance for vocal communication in certain species of songbird (Nottebohm, 1977). In certain of the songbirds which annually learn songs, if appropriate sites in the left hemisphere are lesioned, the birds will fail to learn how to sing, but comparable lesions on the right will have only minor effects. It is probably more than coincidence that, as in man, the strongest subhuman laterality effect is obtained in the control of midline organs used for vocalization.

Nevertheless, although our main concern may be for speech and other kinds of vocal communication, in man there is a related asymmetry in the phenomenon of handedness which is almost as strong as that for speech. Regardless of culture and as far back as the earliest signs of human civilization, the vast majority of people have exhibited marked preferences for one hand or the other (table 6.2). Because it is known that the anatomy of the vocal apparatus of many species – including dogs, monkeys and gorillas is unsuitable for the generation of many of the sounds of human-like speech, perhaps hemispheric asymmetries can be detected in the handedness of animals. Handedness is a phenomenon which we might expect to be more pervasive in the animal world than speech-like activity – as pervasive perhaps as the ability to undertake skilled movements of the hands and feet.

To be sure, whenever an apparent discontinuity in the evolutionary continuum is found, scientists will look for signs of continuity – in this case, signs of handedness in other species. The most intensive empirical search has been for handedness in other mammalian species and it has been a disappointing result for some (e.g. Hamilton, 1977) to find that there is no *species* predilection for left or right hand (paw) usage.

Table 6.2 Handedness in man

Culture	Subjects	Percentage right-handers
Scotland	Children and adults	86.0
Australia	Children	88.0
North America	Children and adults	88.2
Eskimo	Adults	88.7
Australia	Adults	89.5
Greece	Children	89.7
America	Children	90.0
Tonga	Young adults	91.0
Taiwan	Children and adults	94.0
Sweden	Adults	94.6
Japan	Adults	96.9
Solomon Islands	Children and adults	97.2
Hong Kong	Adults	98.5
Congo	Children	99.5

This negative evidence, however, is negative only with regard to the question whether or not there are congenital factors which produce fairly consistent anatomical asymmetries and therefore *species* asymmetries. A far more important issue concerns not population asymmetries, but rather the acquired handedness of individual animals. Here surprisingly the evidence is positive (if its significance remains debatable). As a rule rats, mice, cats, dogs and monkeys *individually* show rather strong preferences for using one hand (paw) or the other for carrying out relatively complex tasks. Moreover, that preference tends to remain for the given task for extended periods of time. Instead of developing a dominant *hemisphere*, however, animals will usually develop highly idiosyncratic patterns of dominance – with one hand favored for one task, the other favored for similar or different tasks. This pattern has been described by Hamilton (1977) as 'ludicrously variable,' but it should be emphasized that the variability (at least for the skilled tasks) is not within a single task, but across tasks. The animals do not develop 'dominant hemispheres,' but they do develop 'dominant engrams' – some of which will be in the left and some in the right hemisphere.

Binocular depth perception and the role of the corpus callosum

A normal sense of depth perception depends crucially upon visual information reaching the cortex from both eyes and making comparisons between the slightly disparate images. As illustrated in figure 6.9, when the eyes focus on an object at a certain distance, those objects which are beyond the point of fixation will be projected to the medial (or nasal) half of the retina in both eyes, and those which are in front of the fixation point will be projected to the lateral (or temporal) half, again in both eyes. The nature of the images coming to the two retinas are, however, slightly different and a comparison of those images provides a means for extracting information concerning the depth of the objects relative to the fixation point. Although, as has been noted, the primary visual cortex has a paucity of callosal fibers, secondary and tertiary visual cortical regions have abundant callosal connections.

In single cell studies using cats and monkeys, neurons which may be involved in depth perception have been identified from the fact that they are driven (excited) by light stimuli to either eye. That the corpus callosum is in fact involved in bilateral responses has been demonstrated by the fact that when the corpus callosum is severed, many such binocularly driven cells become monocularly driven. Payne *et al.* (1984) have shown this phenomenon in the cat. Prior to callosal section, three-quarters of more than 400 cells in visual cortex were binocular, whereas only one-half were so after callosumectomy. The fact that still a relatively large percentage of cells are binocular after the sectioning is likely due to the relatively broad overlapping of the visual images going to both hemispheres of the brain. In man and monkey the

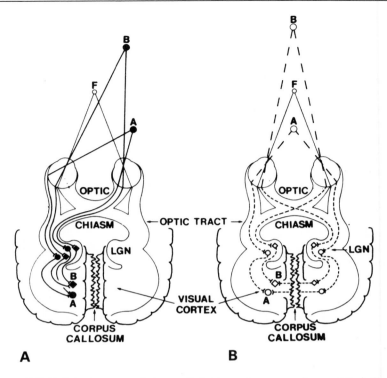

Figure 6.9 Deficits in stereopsis in a split-brain patient, according to Mitchell and Blakemore (1970). Without callosal communication, each hemisphere is capable of making depth judgments for objects away from the midline because all relevant information is sent to one or the other hemisphere (A), but when the objects to be compared fall on the midline, all of the relevant information is not made available to either hemisphere (B), thus requiring the cooperation of the hemispheres.

overlap is confined to only one degree on either side of the vertical midline, but in the cat the overlap is increased to ± 4 degrees. In any event, the incidence of binocularity was significantly reduced by callosal section – a fact suggesting that many cortical cells receive contralateral *excitatory* input across the corpus callosum.

As has often been the case in laterality research, the clearest illustration of hemispheric cooperation in depth perception is to be found in an experiment on one of the split-brain human patients, as studied by Mitchell and Blakemore (1970). Their theoretical argument is depicted in figure 6.9. They reasoned that depth perception which relies on the comparison of disparate images would suffer when the two retinal images were sent to the surgically separated hemispheres (figure 6.9(B)), but not suffer when the two images were sent to the same hemisphere (and thus compared intrahemispherically) (figure 6.9(A)).

Study of this figure will suffice to show that objects which are presented to one side or the other of the midline fixation point will be compared intrahemispherically, whereas those presented in front of or behind the midline fixation point will require callosal mechanisms for comparison.

By asking the commissurotomy patient (LB) to fixate on a center point and then presenting for 100 milliseconds visual stimuli which were located either nearer to or further from the subject than the fixation point. It was found that when the stimuli were 6 degrees to the right of the midline (thus perceived by the language hemisphere), LB had little difficulty in determining the position of the stimulus relative to the fixation point. He was reported to have been confident in his judgments and to have been correct in sixteen out of twenty trials. But when the stimuli were presented on the midline, thus requiring hemispheric coordination, he was found to be 'very restless and uncertain in his judgements.' He was correct in only seven out of twenty trials – a success rate which is not significantly better than chance guessing.

It should be noted that an excitatory 'relay' function of the corpus callosum in depth perception is implicated in this study. Indeed it is hard to imagine an inhibitory mechanism through which the 'comparison of disparate images' could be efficiently accomplished. Similarly callosal fibers connecting primary auditory cortical regions are likely to be excitatory to allow a comparison of the strength of the auditory stimulus reaching both ears. It does not inevitably follow that all callosal functions are excitatory (as advocated by Gazzaniga and LeDoux, 1978), but undoubtedly the clearest example of hemispheric coordination (in-depth perception) implicates an excitatory role.

7

A THEORETICAL FRAMEWORK FOR THE STUDY OF THE BRAIN CODE

In the preceding chapters theoretical arguments and experimental findings concerning the possible inhibitory role of the corpus callosum have been reviewed. The evidence is persuasive, I believe, for considering that at least some portions of association cortex on the left and right have complementary functions – most appropriately summarized in *Homo sapiens* as language and context – *due to inhibitory callosal effects*. In other words it may be that we have identified *one* mechanism of interhemispheric communication in man. If this claim can be sustained, there are various implications for research on brain laterality – but are we justified in speaking of implications for the fundamental nature of the *brain code*?

In order to answer this question, let us return to the earlier discussion of the already deciphered codes of nature. Let us take a closer look at the general features of the atomic code and the genetic code to determine what constitutes truly fundamental mechanisms of information transfer at those levels. We will then be in a position to make some general statements about the possible significance of callosal inhibition for the 'brain code.'

How are natural systems organized?

For several years I have been interested in the functional similarities found among diverse natural systems (Cook, 1980b). My original motivation was simply to come to an understanding of the fundamental features of the atom, cell and human organism, but I eventually realized that there are indeed some general principles of systemic organization which apply regardless of the actual physical system under consideration. Many such cross-level similarities are discussed in the 'general systems theory' literature and provide an unusually coherent context within which to study the natural sciences and the philosophy of science (Laszlo, 1973). For me, however, the most fascinating aspect of systems thinking has been the similarities of control mechanisms among vastly different natural, social and cybernetic systems. Specifically the fact that each of the three most fundamental natural systems known to science – the atom, the cell and the animal organism – makes use of a dual control structure seems to be an important principle of natural organization. The dualities in these systems are now well-known aspects of empirical science, but their significance as a general principle of systemic organization is not widely appreciated.

The duality of the brain – and perhaps the mind – has been a recurring topic of serious study and popular speculation for well over 100 years (Harrington, 1986). Although strictly speaking scientific advances in this realm have been infrequent, a wide range of empirical findings in normal and abnormal psychology has been related to differences in function of the cerebral hemispheres. Because the hemispheres are normally linked to one another via the forebrain commissures and – in any case – receive virtually identical sensory stimuli, major conflicts between the two sides would seem unlikely. Nevertheless bilaterally symmetrical nervous systems can in some respects be considered as two heavily interconnected, but complete and self-sufficient entities – with virtually the full range of sensory, associative and motor components required for 'normal' functioning. Only when the commissures are cut, however, does their independence become blatant. The most interesting such case is that of a patient referred to as P.S. who, when asked what his intended profession is, wrote 'draftsman' with the staid left hemisphere and 'racing car driver' with the sporting right hemisphere! P.S. has neither a typical brain nor a typical split-brain, but even one such case suggests that the two halves of the brain may be the source of some of the deep internal conflicts which we all experience and which continue to provide fodder for theories of the human psyche. The duality of the brain is an anatomical truism and the duality of mind must therefore be considered as a reasonable hypothesis to pursue.

The duality of cellular control, as embodied in the two forms of nucleic acid, has been apparent since the late 1950s and its fundamental nature is well known, if commented on but rarely. Waddington (1970) is one who has emphasized the importance of this duality:

At the core of the [cellular] system is DNA, a substance which is sufficiently inert and unreactive to serve as a reliable memory store. By itself, it can do almost nothing. . . . However, it occurs in association with enzymes, which in the first place enable it to be replicated, so that there are copies to pass to daughter cells, and which also use the information stored in the DNA to produce a corresponding RNA and that in turn is used to guide the synthesis of a corresponding protein. The whole system works extremely efficiently, but as you can see it involves separating the function of reliability in storing information from that of actually using the information as instructions to change the surroundings. It is, I suppose, theoretically possible to imagine a substance which [is] both inactive enough to be reliable and active enough to have effects in producing a phenotype. Possibly some evolving systems on Mars or elsewhere in the universe have discovered such a perfect answer to the evolutionary problem, but life on earth has not. It is stuck with a system in which there is an inescapable difference between the genotype – what is transmitted, the DNA – and the phenotype – what is produced when the genotype is used as instructions [the RNA].

Conceivably cells could be regulated elsewise and 'the evolutionary problem' resolved in other ways, but currently no viable alternative means for maintaining secure information storage and for allowing effective information usage is known in cell science – suggesting that the control duality is not only useful, but perhaps essential to life processes.

In the atom there is again a fundamental duality in the atomic nucleus where the nucleons exist in two distinct forms, protons and neutrons. Physicists rarely comment upon this duality, but its importance is implicit to the spectrum of stable isotopes across the periodic chart. That is approximately equal numbers of protons and neutrons are required in all atoms to achieve nuclear stability and atomic species are simply and accurately characterized by the numbers of each kind of nucleon present. Again theoretical arguments might suggest the existence of proton-less or neutron-less nuclei, but in fact the natural world demands an approximate balance in the number of each type of nucleon in the nucleus of any atom.

In rebuttal couldn't it be argued that spurious dichotomies come cheap and usually lead nowhere? Perhaps we could as easily dream up trichotomies or other overly simplistic schema for classification and somehow force all natural phenomena into them as well? There would undoubtedly be no harm in searching for other cross-level patterns in nature, but it is unlikely that other schema could be devised without demanding that much of natural science also be rewritten! Quite independently and without the influences of 'cross-disciplinary' thinking, physicists have discovered that atomic nuclei have two kinds of nucleons in their nuclei, biologists have shown that two kinds of nucleic acid govern cellular functions, and psychologists, zoologists and others have found that virtually all animal nervous systems have bilateral control.

In other words, there are in fact some unusual features of the control dichotomies in the atom, cell and animal organisms which make them fundamental. The two control elements at each level are nearly identical – certainly far more similar to each other than any other pair of regulatory components in those systems. So we can say that we have not arbitrarily pulled out any set of objects in order to satisfy some preconceived notion of dual control. More importantly the two control elements are the most fundamental 'informational' structures in these systems. Cells don't just happen to have DNA in them; they are run by DNA, using RNA messengers. Similarly, among the plethora of ephemeral elementary particles within the atom, the primary factor which decides the character of the atom is the amount of nuclear charge

182

– which, in turn, is a direct consequence of the balance of nuclear protons and neutrons. At least with regard to the human organism (and no matter what Plato may have thought), people are run by their brains and, no matter how mute the right hemisphere may be, both halves appear to be essential for normal, high-level cognition. Other species probably utilize *both* sides of their brains for their characteristically high-level cognition and complex motor activity.

So let us make no compromises on this point! Control dualities are a fundamental aspect of the regulation of at least the three principal entities in the known physical, biological and psychological worlds. Some pointless nit-picking could be indulged in (the abundant, but neutron-less hydrogen atom; the abundant, but DNA-less viruses; the nearly normal hemispherectomy patients, etc.), but, for the skeptic, the validity of this assertion concerning the importance in nature of dual control structures can be tested quite easily by asking any physicist, biologist or psychologist what the 'basic pieces' in his field are. If you can get the physicist to step back from his current research interests for a moment, he will probably outline the 'central dogma' of atomic physics (without using that phrase):

$$\text{Neutrons} \longleftrightarrow \text{Protons} \rightarrow \text{Electrons}$$

The biologist will triumphantly outline his 'central dogma' (and will invariably use that phrase):

$$\text{DNA} \longleftrightarrow \text{RNA} \rightarrow \text{Proteins}$$

The psychologist will probably take more time coming up with something clear-cut, so if you prompt him with some questions about the most firmly established aspects of human neuropsychology, the role of the forebrain commissures, the nature of cerebral laterality, etc. his answers will probably be consistent with a schema concerning high-level information processing (which he will definitely *not* call a 'central dogma'), such as:

$$\text{Right hemisphere} \longleftrightarrow \text{Left hemisphere} \rightarrow \text{Somatic structure}$$
$$\text{(dominant hand and organs of speech)}$$

There can consequently be little doubt that there are at least some first-order structural similarities among these diverse systems, but what about functional similarities? Is there an underlying principle of systemic functioning which requires dual control? As I have argued in a previous book (Cook, 1980b), I believe a strong case can be made for considering that dual control structures allow these systems to maintain informational stability over extended periods of time and yet simultaneously to remain flexible enough to interact with their environments.

183

Because the material composition of these systems is so diverse, the exact nature of the balance between internal control (or 'stability') and external control (or 'flexibility') varies widely. Nevertheless, despite differences in the means for attaining similar goals – it is not unreasonable to suspect that some such balance between systemic constancy and informational continuity, on the one hand, and systemic fluidity and the ability to give and take with the external world, on the other, must be attained. Stability is required in order that the system can preserve an identity within a necessarily fluctuating and potentially disruptive environment; flexibility is required in order that the needs of the system can be met and the system itself can make appropriate responses to its environment. By employing virtually identical subcomponents to perform these contrasting functions, it appears that an inherent balance between these two tendencies is achieved. Importantly the usage of two structurally similar elements will ensure that they will be able to communicate with one another in the same language. By means of complementary specializations of two similar elements for (i) internal control and (ii) external control, systems of this particular design embody an inherent balance between tendencies toward preservation of the current informational content of the system and, contrarily, toward its usage and alteration. Due therefore to the advantages which such balance confers, it is conceivable that systems constructed in this way have – as a consequence – fared well in the natural selection of material entities at the respective levels of material complexity, in comparison with various other theoretically possible systems which embody other forms of internal organization.

Detailed argument concerning this isomorphism would take us too far astray at this point (see Laszlo's *Introduction to General Systems Philosophy*, 1973, for an introduction to this field and my own book, *Stability and Flexibility*, 1980b, for further details on control dualities). Suffice it to say that there are some intriguing similarities among diverse natural systems, which the psychologist could do worse than to examine. In the present context we are concerned primarily with placing our detailed knowledge of the brain within a much larger theoretical framework – specifically within the broad framework of evolution. The danger of any such theoretical perspective is that we may be led astray – either (i) following, for example, an abstract 'input–black box–output' model which, even if in some sense valid, simply cannot be translated into the unambiguous language of scientific neuropsychology, or (ii) following a specific and concrete model which then leads us, for example, to search for computer paraphernalia which simply don't exist in living brains. In other words we may be seduced into abstract philosophy or mathematics and never return to genuine psychology, or we may become so impressed with some well-understood physical system or biological entity that we end up perceiving all of the findings of neuroscience in terms of that particular system.

On the other hand, if we remain within an evolutionary context and ask questions about why various systems are constructed as they are, general principles of organization may become apparent. Judicious use of analogies with other systems may help us to reorganize our knowledge of the brain into useful categories and help us to perceive the human organism as one of a fairly small number of very successful natural systems. Particularly in the case of biological systems, precise knowledge concerning both structure and function is often available, and some explicit lessons are there to be learned about the natural selection of viable systems. The relevance of atomic physics for brain science is not immediately obvious, but again we have available to us a natural system, the basic features of which are well understood and not terribly complex. Quite simply, there may be some heuristic benefits in perusing the successes of quantum physics and molecular biology when trying to put the diverse findings concerning the brain into a sensible theoretical framework. That, at any rate, is the optimistic justification for pursuing in the present chapter the above-mentioned analogies with other well-known systems.

I do not argue that any similarities with other systems can alter our core conclusions about the brain, and specifically the role of the corpus callosum, as discussed in chapters 1–6; on the contrary the psychological arguments must stand on their own. Isomorphism with other systems might, however, lead us to conclusions concerning the *significance* of, for example, callosal function for our understanding of brain processes or might suggest a hierarchy of importance for the established facts. In an extremely anti-theoretical vein, it would perhaps be possible to accept all of the individual conclusions of chapters 1–6 and yet reject all implications for the nature of the brain code. Indeed there may be those who would be reluctant to bring into the already complex discussion on brain function issues which are not directly and unavoidably relevant. Nevertheless, the broader theoretical context could be instructive and, at worst, will be inappropriate.

Particularly in light of the continuing temptation for some physiologists to resolve questions concerning human free-will, the mind–body problem, etc., in terms of Heisenberg's uncertainty principle (which is itself a quagmire of philosophical problems),[1] a healthy skepticism

---

[1] M. Bunge's *Metascientific Inquiries* (1959) remains the best exposition of the various and yet unresolved problems raised by the uncertainty principle. While many physicists implicitly accept the 'Copenhagen' or indeterminist interpretation of the uncertainty principle – i.e. that there is an inherent uncertainty *in nature* (a nano-second of free-will!), such a view is not an inevitable consequence of the mathematical expression of uncertainty and has been vigorously opposed by many of the big guns in theoretical physics (including Einstein, Schrodinger, Planck, deBroglie and Lande). Even if we were to accept the empirical validity of 'uncertainty' (that, for example, the position and the momentum of a particle cannot be *measured* with unlimited precision), it remains a controversial question whether or not the particle itself at any given moment *has* precise position and momentum. Until the debate is resolved at the level of particle physics, it would seem unwise for the physiologist to set up any chosen interpretation of uncertainty as the cornerstone of a theory of the brain!

concerning the particle physicist's potential contribution to brain science is fully warranted. Yet it is worth emphasizing that making use of concepts from atomic physics does not necessarily imply a crude reductionism; on the contrary, rather than insisting that a phenomenon at one level invades and determines phenomena at other levels, we might be able to make use of concepts in well-understood fields when exploring less well-understood areas.

Moreover I suspect that some of the old hands in psychology who have chased rats through multifarious mazes and ablated monkeys into multifarious neurological deficits may have long ago concluded that the complexity of the brain simply precludes the possibility of a fundamental 'code' – comparable, say, to the molecular biologist's nucleotide base-pairing. The pessimists may, of course, be correct, but their negative view is patently the voice of failure – *either* because there is no code to be discovered *or* because no one had discovered the forest amidst the dendritic trees. So, wary of some of the possible pitfalls and wary of the possible non-existence of a brain code, let us examine more closely the atomic and cellular systems in search of general principles of systemic organization.

THE ATOMIC SYSTEM

A dichotomy of control is most easily seen in the atomic system, which is regulated by the two forms of nucleon, the proton and neutron (figure 7.1). In most respects they are virtually identical (table 7.1), but only the proton has a net electrostatic charge and consequently it alone interacts with the electrons in its atomic and molecular environment. The neutron is electrostatically neutral and therefore has virtually no effect on and is virtually unaffected by the surrounding electromagnetic milieu, but it has a central role in maintaining the stability of the nucleus itself. Without such neutral particles present to bind the mutually repelling protons, the nucleus would explode and the long-term stability of the atomic system would be impossible.

For many intelligent people (including some psychologists), words like atom, neutron, electron and molecule imply the same thing: extremely small (and therefore irrelevant to everyday life). As illustrated in figure 7.1, however, the isolated atom is the smallest and simplest complete system known to science and may have some heuristic value even to those of us worried primarily about multibillion atom entities, such as brains and people. The atom has an internal structure and can be seen to embody some rather interesting principles of self-organization. The positive charge in the nucleus ranges from 1 to about 100 units; depending upon the size of that central charge, the atom will be capable of attracting and holding a comparable number of negatively charged electrons – either on its own as an isolated atom or ion, or sharing electrons with other atoms within a large molecule or crystal.

Table 7.1 The major features of the nucleons

	Neutron	Proton
Similarities		
Electromagnetic radius	0.8×10^{-15} m	0.8×10^{-15} m
Mass	1.6727×10^{-27} kg	1.6749×10^{-27} kg
Angular momentum	½	½
Parity	+	+
Subcomponents	quarks (?)	quarks (?)
Dissimilarities		
Net charge	0	+1
Magnetic moment	−1.91 nuclear magnetons	+2.79 nuclear magnetons
Stability	7.2×10^3 sec	infinite (?)

Table 7.2 The major features of the nucleic acids

	DNA	RNA
Constituent molecules	D-deoxyribose phosphate nucleotide bases adenine guanine cytosine thymine	D-ribose phosphate nucleotide bases adenine guanine cytosine uracil (various modifications of the above bases)
Functional unit	nucleotide base	nucleotide base
Informational content	Dependent upon linear sequence of nucleotide bases	Dependent upon linear sequence of nucleotide bases
Molecular weight	4–15 million Daltons	20,000–1,000,000 Daltons

Since the positively charged protons are tightly packed within the nucleus, there is a tremendous repulsive force between neighboring protons – amounting to almost 1 million times the electrostatic force with which an electron is attracted to a proton. For this reason, nuclear stability requires the presence of non-repulsive neutral particles within the nucleus, i.e. neutrons. The neutrons bind to one another and to protons without contributing to the internal repulsion of the nucleus,

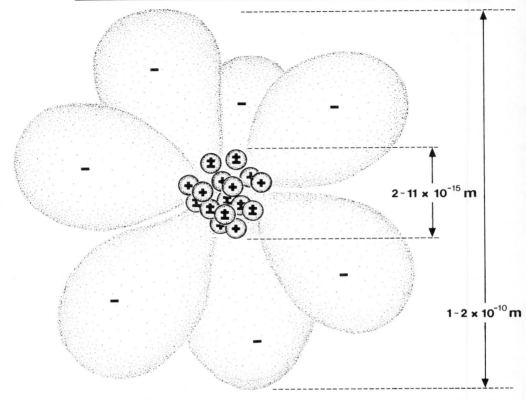

$2 \sim 11 \times 10^{-15}$ m

$1 \sim 2 \times 10^{-10}$ m

Figure 7.1 The atomic system. Within the nucleus there are positively charged protons and neutral neutrons. The negatively charged electron configuration is held around the nucleus by the proton's positive electrostatic charge. Despite their strong mutual electrostatic repulsion, the protons are held within the nucleus due to the stronger, even attractive nuclear force acting among protons and neutrons. The neutrons serve as an important nuclear 'glue.'

and thereby allow for the existence of stable nuclei containing more than one proton. Curiously, isolated neutrons are themselves unstable and break down into a proton, an electron and other bits and pieces, unless they are within a nucleus with a sufficient number of protons.

When an appropriate balance of protons and neutrons is reached, the neutrons act to hold the nucleus together and to maintain a constant nuclear charge – thus producing a stable atom with characteristic properties. Unlike neutrons, protons are stable particles – participating in the electromagnetic exchange of photons with peripheral electrons and consequently maintaining continual contact with the atom's external reality. There are in fact small magnetic and gravitational interactions between the neutron and the electron, but the magnitude of those forces is only a fraction of 1 percent of the electrostatic interaction between proton and electron. In our first-order approximation of the atomic system, it is therefore reasonable to say that the neutron is concerned solely with nuclear activities, whereas the proton is concerned heavily with peripheral (atomic and molecular) events.

THE CELLULAR SYSTEM

In the living cell there is a well-known division of labor between the two forms of nucleic acid, DNA and RNA (figure 7.2). In most respects DNA and RNA are structurally very similar – so much so that, given the raw materials and appropriate enzymes, a DNA molecule can construct an RNA molecule (the so-called 'transcription' process) or an RNA molecule can construct a DNA molecule ('reverse transcription').

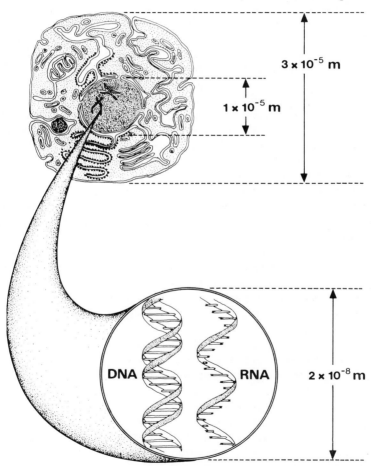

3×10^{-5} m

1×10^{-5} m

DNA RNA

2×10^{-8} m

Figure 7.2 The cellular system. Within the cellular nucleus are found the majority of the nucleic acids, DNA and RNA. Most DNA remains within the nuclear membrane rather than venturing into the metabolically dangerous cytoplasm, whereas much of the RNA enters the cytoplasm where it translates the nucleic acid information into protein form.

189

There are, in fact, a number of small structural differences between the nucleic acids (table 7.2) – which undoubtedly play a role in determining their functional differences. Like the proton in the atomic system, the RNA seems to do all of the essential 'work' of the cellular system in translating the genetic information into functional protein molecules (the 'translation' process) in the cellular cytoplasm. Like the atom's nuclear neutrons, the DNA is essential for the long-term preservation of the system as a whole and for the temporal continuity of its genetic information. Since RNA molecules are often destroyed in the biologically active cytoplasm, maintenance of the character of the given cell depends crucially on the ability of the DNA to remain unaltered within the cellular nucleus and there to transcribe RNA molecules – to reassert its genetic message in the cytoplasm through the repeated construction of RNA molecules. Although the nature of the information involved in the living cell appears to be vastly more complex than that in the non-living atom and although the structure of the cell is vastly different from that of the atom, it is evident that, as in the atomic system, one control element (the RNA) exerts immediate effects on the surrounding peripheral structure of the system (the cellular cytoplasm and its wider environment), while the other control element (the DNA) has primarily internal 'nuclear' control – maintaining the system as a coherent whole over extended periods of time.

Realizing that specialization is an essential part of the scientific endeavor, it is remarkable that these very general principles of natural organization are not explicitly a part of early school education. Although there may be good reason to believe that the real-world relevance of atomic structure lies primarily in its implications for nuclear energy and electron flow in semiconductors and athough there may be good practical reasons to emphasize the biotechnological impact of the DNA–RNA story, nonetheless conceptually there are some simple and arguably far more important lessons to be learned about how the preeminent systems in the known universe work! When viewed from this perspective, not only is modern science technologically competent and worth knowing about for its material benefits, but also it is conceptually profound and intrinsically interesting – regardless of how we may choose to apply that knowledge.

THE ANIMAL ORGANISM

At the next level of natural organization, this principle of dual control is most clearly seen in terms of the dynamics of the human organism, but the principle appears to hold true for all mammalian species and perhaps for all animal organisms with bilateral nervous systems. In human neuropsychology it is well established that one cerebral hemisphere, normally the left, is involved in the control of the organs of speech and the favored hand (figure 7.3). The fact of left-hemispheric dominance for the control of the *quintessentially human* motor activities – speech

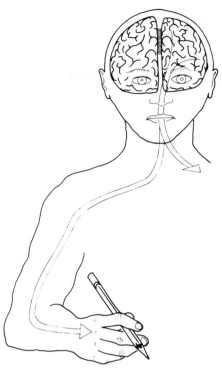

Figure 7.3 The human organism. Despite approximate bilateral symmetry of the brain, the quintessentially *human* effects on the social and natural world are brought about through speech and tool-making predominantly by the left hemisphere. It is the 'executive' side of the brain, but is connected some 200 million times to its 'board of directors' on the right.

and tool-making – indicates a functional dichotomy which is truly fundamental.

Right-hemispheric control is found in a small minority of left-handers, but bilateral control is unusual and may be a source of early learning disabilities and stuttering (e.g. Zimmerman and Knott, 1974). For whatever reasons, it is apparent that cerebral *asymmetry* of function has been selected in the evolution of man. It is perhaps less clear what the unique talents of the right hemisphere may be (see chapters 4 and 5), but insofar as reading, writing, speech production, speech comprehension and tool-making are controlled predominantly by the left hemisphere, it is certain that the right hemisphere has minimal 'external control' capacities (except under unusual circumstances such as subsequent to callosal transection or left-hemispheric damage).

The structural differences between the left and right hemispheres were reviewed in chapter 4 and are summarized in table 7.3. As was the case in the cellular specializations of RNA and DNA, the innate

Table 7.3 Anatomical asymmetries of the cerebral hemispheres in man

Region	Finding	Reference
Planum temporale	left > right	Geschwind and Levitsky (1968)
Hemisphere weight	right > left	LeMay (1976)
Broca's area	right > left	Wada et al. (1975)
Subcortical regions	more white matter in right hemisphere than left	Gur et al. (1983)
Occipital lobe	left > right	LeMay (1976)
Neurotransmitters	more epinephrine in left hemisphere than right	Oke et al. (1978)
	more serotonin in right hemisphere than left	Mandell and Knapp (1979)
Corticopyramidal tract	left hemisphere contribution to right pyramidal tract is greater than vice versa	Flor-Henry (1983)
Sylvian fissure length	left > right	LeMay and Culebras (1972)

functional differences of the cerebral hemispheres found in newborn children must be a complex result of small structural differences – but, as with RNA and DNA, those functional specializations should not obscure our appreciation of the fundamental similarities. The cerebral hemispheres are so alike that damage to either in early life will lead eventually to nearly normal behavior – with the intact hemisphere assuming the duties normally carried out on the other side. And yet in the normal brain, it is usually the case that the left hemisphere is the 'talker' and the 'doer,' while the right hemisphere plays an important cognitive role in putting the left hemisphere's activities within their proper contexts.

If indeed the right hemisphere is involved virtually full time with the processing of high-level 'contextual' information – comparable to that made explicit through language by the left hemisphere, then the flow of information in the typical atomic, cellular and human organismic systems can be summarized by three versions of 'central dogma' at the three levels of organization (Cook 1980b):

$$\text{Neutron} \longleftrightarrow \text{Proton} \rightarrow \text{Electron}$$

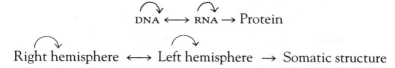

The generality of this pattern of information flow in animal species other than man is somewhat problematical, but two important facts suggest similar specialization in other bilateral nervous systems. In the only other species known to communicate complex information via the vocal chords (as distinct from the instinctual calls of many species), i.e. in the songbirds, the left hemisphere is again dominant, with little or no capacity of the right hemisphere to learn or generate specific song patterns (Nottebohm, 1977). Secondly, although congenital 'dominance' in other mammalian species remains a controversial issue, it is well established that the vast majority of rodents, cats, dogs and non-human primates which are trained to perform *complex* motor tasks develop a favored paw or hand (e.g. Collins, 1977; Warren, 1977; Webster, 1977) (see chapter 6). Such unilateral 'dominance' of one hemisphere persists over time for the given task. There is in fact no left or right predominance within the species as a whole, but individual animals normally show clear dominance: one cerebral hemisphere assumes the role of 'executive' for a given task, while the other hemisphere, with presumably nearly identical neural hardware, functions elsewise.

In other words, although there is considerable bilateral structural symmetry of the animal brain and, in mammals, extensive communication between the two halves via the forebrain commissures, only one of the two cerebral hemispheres normally develops the necessary engrams to perform a given complex task. Unless there is some prior anatomical factor which biases the system toward left- or right-sided dominance (as is apparently the case in man and the songbirds), the dominance of one hand or paw may result from random influences and chance events – such as which hand/paw was used in the first successful attempt at performing the task – rather than any intrinsic neuronal advantage. Whatever the mechanism of dominance, a continued advantage on one side would likely result from the inhibition of the contralateral hemisphere – resulting in the 'handedness' of most animals. It follows that early transection of the corpus callosum in animals would reduce the incidence of strong left- or right-handedness. Provided that the effects of practice can be controlled, greater bilateralization would be predicted.

Although it is unclear what the 'non-dominant' hemisphere is doing in subhuman forms, by virtue of homotopic commissural connections, the contralateral hemisphere inevitably would have patterns of neural activity which are in some way complementary to those of the 'dominant' hemisphere.

Whether or not it makes sense to speak of the 'context' of a motor skill (in the sense developed in chapter 4) is uncertain, but – aside from cognitive implications – homotopic callosal inhibition would imply that the 'dominant' motor engram would be stored in a different (i.e. not directly utilizable) form, but its inversion across the corpus callosum would reproduce the original engram. In other words the specific motor activity could be initiated from either hemisphere, but successful realization of the motor skill would require working via the engram of the dominant hemisphere. For this reason, it is thought likely that the 'central dogma' of human neuropsychology applies to all mammalian brains (although the side of the executive 'dominance' may vary with the individual animal and with the specific task). In other words, while one hemisphere is dominant for executive control of the animal's somatic structure during any given skilled activity, the other hemisphere is involved with storage of complementary information, which itself cannot be used for motor activity, but which might be used to trigger the motor activity guided by the dominant hemisphere.

If it can be concluded that the 'non-dominant' hemisphere in man and other species stores information which is complementary to the 'dominant' motor engrams, then it can be said that the three predominant systems in the physical, biological and psychological realms have evolved with 'dual control mechanisms' in which one of two nearly identical regulatory components is 'externally oriented,' whereas the other is 'internally oriented' (see table 7.4) – communicating with the external control element, but not capable of external control functions.

To recapitulate, the first-order description of any atom requires knowledge of the number of protons (to specify the element), the number of neutrons (to specify the isotope), and peripherally the number of electrons (to specify the ion). While various other particles are involved in the interactions of these three important classes of particle, knowledge concerning only the nucleons and electrons is required for an understanding of the physicochemical properties of any given atomic system.

Cells can be similarly characterized solely in terms of the three types of informational macromolecule. The DNA content of a cell specifies the individual organism, the RNA content specifies its differentiated state (as neuron, liver cell, etc.) and its protein content specifies its actual level of activity – the current differentiated status of the cell. As important as carbohydrates, lipids, fats and the other organic and inorganic molecules of the cell may be, a fundamental understanding of a given cellular system depends primarily on knowledge of the nature and activity of its informational molecules – which ultimately regulate all other molecular events in the cell.

Finally, with regard to the 'central dogma' of human neuropsychology, our current understanding of the brain forces us to acknowledge that the cognitive and effective contents of individual minds are

Table 7.4 Isomorphic control structures in various natural systems

Level of natural organization	Control center	Internal control element	External control element	Peripheral structure	Academic discipline	Central dogma
Subatomic particles	*	*	*	*	Particle physics	*
Atom	Nucleus	Neutron	Proton	Electron	Atomic physics	Yes
Molecule	*	*	*	*	Chemistry	*
Cell	Nucleus	DNA	RNA	Protein	Molecular biology	Yes
Tissue	*	*	*	*	Histology	*
Organ	*	*	*	*	Histology	*
Plant organism	*	*	*	*	Botany	*
Animal organism	Brain	'Non-dominant' hemisphere	'Dominant' hemisphere	Somatic structure	Neurosciences	(See text)
Higher-level systems	.	.	.	.	.	.
	.	.	.	.	.	.
	.	.	.	.	.	.

Note: * non-existent or unknown.

integrated and controlled in a complex way by the two cerebral hemispheres – not primarily by the lower brainstem or peripheral somatic structures. Furthermore realization of the needs and desires of individual minds in the social world is brought about primarily by the control of peripheral 'effector mechanisms' (the organs of speech and the skilled movements of peripheral musculature) through the workings of predominantly the left cerebral hemisphere. This is not by any means to assert that structures other than the cerebral cortex are irrelevant to the shape of personality, but the integration of all information and the final decision-making processes are likely to occur at a cortical level – and ultimately to utilize a final common pathway through the left hemisphere in the control of somatic motor mechanisms.

It may not be possible to 'characterize' people as neatly and as succinctly as it is possible to characterize atoms and cells, but it necessarily follows that a first-order personality theory should be based upon quantification of the control center elements, i.e. (i) the executive 'talents' of the left hemisphere, (ii) the conceptual/contextual framework of the right hemisphere, and (iii) the balance between the two realms.

Something akin to Eysenck's extroversion–introversion dimension or perhaps a simple tabulation of the individual's technical skills might be a sufficient measure of left-hemispheric activation. Something akin to Eysenck's neuroticism–stability dimension might reflect the degree of left–right balance (or the degree to which one's daily activities are in agreement with one's system of beliefs), but an independent measure of the nature of the conceptual framework in the right hemisphere has apparently not been devised. Clearly such a measure would have more of a psychoanalytic flavor to it than the behavioristic measures suitable for evaluating the left hemisphere, but some measure of the larger conceptual issues which underlie human personalities would seem essential to quantify the strength of right-hemisphere activity. Perhaps some of the current personality measures of emotional lability, impulsiveness, etc., could serve as indirect indices of right-hemisphere activity, but it is worth noting that they focus on behavior – where the left hemisphere plays such an important role, rather than on the right hemisphere's 'nuclear' role.

Known and potential characterizations of these systems are summarized in table 7.5.

The atomic code and the genetic code

At the very least there are some intriguing structural and functional similarities among the atom, cell and human organism, but are there similarities in the mechanisms of internal communication? First, let us consider the nature of information transmission in the cellular system. The transcription of genetic information from DNA to RNA molecules

Table 7.5 Characterizations of the principal systems of nature

System	Characterization of the system in terms of:			
	Internal control structure	External control structure	Balance between internal and external control	Peripheral structure
Atom	Isotope	Element	Nuclear stability/ instability	Chemical status
Cell	Species	Cell type (i.e. differentiated state)	Potential for further differentiation	Metabolic status
Human organism	Motivations	Talents	Social mobility	Social status

involves the pairing of stereochemically complementary nucleotide bases (figure 7.4). For a given purine or pyrimidine base in a DNA chain, there is an RNA pyrimidine or purine base which can bind to its DNA complement through hydrogen bonds. This 'negation' of the molecular information of the DNA imples that the RNA contains *not* information identical to that in the DNA, but information which is its complement or 'negative.' Only through a second transfer process will the original molecular information be retrieved. It is important to note, however, that transcription entails a second type of inversion of the molecular information. That is due to the directionality of the nucleic acids (as they are read by enzymes from the 5' to the 3' end), the molecular information which is passed from DNA to RNA is not only negated into a complementary sequence of purines and pyrimidines, but is also completely reversed end-to-end. If the segment of DNA is a sequence of nucleotide bases such as AGCTTC, then the transcribed RNA would become GAAGCU. In other words, the transfer of genetic information from DNA to RNA or vice versa requires its *double* inversion.

Despite the similarity of a structural duality of control in the atom, it is not obvious on *a priori* grounds that the interaction between the control elements in the atomic system would be isomorphic with the interaction between the isomorphic control center elements of the living cell, but indeed an isomorphic interaction appears to take place. The 'information' of a nucleon can be stored in only two forms: (i) in the temporo-spatial configuration of its mass and (ii) in the temporo-spatial configuration of its charge. All nucleonic properties (angular momentum, magnetic moment, parity, etc.) can ultimately be described in terms of these fundamental properties of mass and charge. It is of considerable interest therefore that the proton–neutron interaction involves 'inversions' of both the nucleon's mass and charge properties.

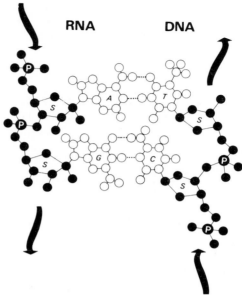

Figure 7.4 Nucleic acid information exchanges. When information is passed from RNA to DNA, or vice versa, the stereochemical pairing of adenine (A) and thymine (T) and that of guanine (G) and cytosine (C) produces a complementary nucleic acid, rather than an exact duplicate. Since the enzymes which pass along RNA or DNA must do so by starting on the so-called 5-prime end of the sugar (S)–phosphate (P) backbone, the newly constructed 'complementary' nucleic acid is, moreover, read 'backwards.' In the example of the figure, the RNA AG sequence has been transcribed into CT. A second transfer would reproduce the original sequence.

As in the cellular system, the most obvious transformation involves nucleonic 'negation.' When neutrons and protons interact through the so-called 'strong' nuclear force, a charged meson is transferred from nucleon to nucleon – resulting in the transformation of a proton into a neutron ($p + pi^- \rightarrow n$) or of a neutron into a proton ($n + pi^+ \rightarrow p$). In order to conserve parity, however, there is a second transformation: the reversal of the nucleon's intrinsic spin. In other words, the movement of the nucleon's mass is thrown into reverse and the nucleon is in effect 'flipped over' (e.g. Enge, 1966; Segre, 1977) into the mirror-image of its original state (see figure 7.5). The nucleon can of course be retrieved in its original configuration of mass and charge by means of a second charged meson transfer, analogous to the recovery of a nucleic acid by means of a second transcription process.

The brain code

As has been discussed in detail in earlier chapters, a hybrid hypothesis which combines elements of both of the prevailing views of callosal function appears to account for many of the central findings of cerebral

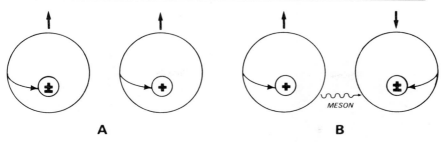

Figure 7.5 Meson exchanges between protons and neutrons. (A) When a neutron and proton interact by means of a negative meson transfer, the charge on the recipient proton is neutralized, while the loss of the neutron's negative charge transforms it into a proton. (B) To conserve parity, one of the two nucleons must undergo a reversal of angular momentum (spin 'up' to spin 'down', or vice versa). A second transfer returns the nucleons to condition A.

laterality research. That is, the topographical inhibitory theory of callosal function (i) is consistent with the main empirical facts concerning brain anatomy and physiology and (ii) implies complementary functioning of the cerebral hemispheres which is not found in either the excitatory hypothesis or the diffuse inhibitory hypothesis. Moreover, the 'complementarity' of the cerebral hemispheres can be shown to be curiously isomorphic with the mechanisms of information transfer in the atomic and cellular systems.

Specifically homotopic callosal inhibition implies two forms of inversion of the neural information as its passes from side-to-side. The transfer of a pattern of neural information from one site on the cortex to any other site over parallel fibers which maintain their relative positions necessarily results in the mirror-image reversal of that information. Assuming no degeneration of the pattern as it is transferred, a pattern identical to the original one would be reproduced by a second mirror-image relay. Such mirror-image relay, however, assumes excitatory connections between the two areas of cortex. If, on the other hand, the nerve fibers have inhibitory effects at their sites of termination, then there would be mirror-image reversal, but also the suppression of the pattern which was activated at the original cortical region.

As such, this mechanism of callosal function is similar to the diffuse inhibitory theory. Inhibition would transfer no information to a region of totally inactive cortex. If, however, the two regions which are involved in this transfer of cortical patterns are both 'aroused' by subcortical mechanisms, then the second area will be the *mirror-image negative* of the first – a pattern of inhibition against a region of increased arousal, the focus of attention (see chapter 4). Without subcortical arousal effects, the second area would have a mirror-image suppression of the original pattern, but suppression against only a region of background activity (figure 3.10d). Stated differently, the greater the arousal of two separate cortical regions which are joined by topographical

LEFT   RIGHT

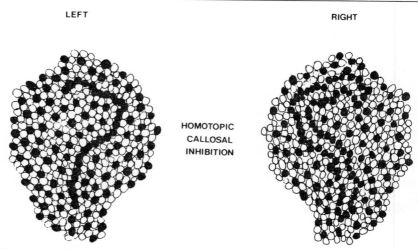

HOMOTOPIC
CALLOSAL
INHIBITION

Figure 7.6 The proposed mechanism for interhemispheric communication. On the left is shown an arbitrary configuration of active cortical columns. On the right is shown the cortical consequence of topographical callosal inhibition. Only topographical *inhibition* produces a double inversion of the pattern on the left.

association fibers, the clearer will be the photographic 'negative' relationship between them.

This mechanism of mirror-image negative mapping between cortical areas could theoretically occur between any two cortical regions with the appropriate anatomical connections between them. It is most likely to occur *inter*hemispherically, however, because of the approximate bilateral symmetry of arousal effects. An identical mechanism of information transfer could be at work *intra*hemispherically between any two cortical regions (with appropriate association fibers) which are aroused simultaneously. For this reason, the interhemispheric process is thought to be one particularly important example of inhibitory cortico-cortical communications in general. In other words, the unusual implications concerning lateral specialization aside, the mirror-image negative mechanism of information transfer may be a fundamental mechanism of information transmission in the brain – a fundamental part of the 'brain code.'

As illustrated in figure 7.7, the control dichotomies in these elementary systems of modern science 'communicate' by means of the double inversion of their information.

In summary, there are some striking analogies among the principal natural systems in terms of structure, function and information flow. Presumably the guiding hand which has produced this recurring theme in the evolution of matter is, broadly defined, natural selection. While no control structure is inevitable or preordained, optimal solutions to the simultaneous demands of systemic continuity and constancy in a

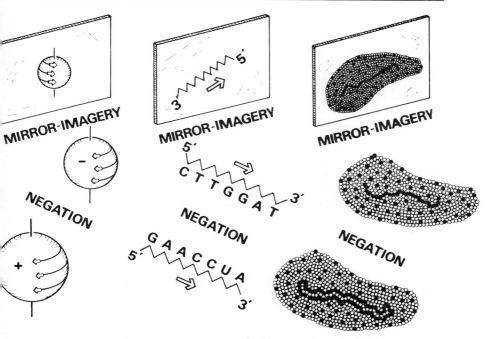

Figure 7.7 The double inversion of information in the atom, cell and animal brain.

changing environment, on the one hand, and systemic flexibility and interaction with the external world, on the other, at each level of material complexity lead, it would appear, to isomorphic mechanisms of information flow.

Systemic pathology

In normal or abnormal situations where arousal is *not* bilaterally symmetrical, the transfer of information between the cerebral hemispheres by means of this mechanism would be decreased or perhaps absent. Although only tangential to this discussion of the brain code, we can be certain that conditions such as schizophrenia represent states in which the fundamental rules of information transfer are in some way disturbed – such that the normal flow of thought is invaded by extraneous thoughts or short-circuited to prevent normal associations. Systematic irregularities in such states may therefore provide further insight into normal functions.

Of particular interest in this regard is the characterization of schizophrenia as a 'partial deconnection syndrome' (Dimond, 1979b) – meaning a condition of impaired callosal transfer between the cerebral hemispheres. Unlike the normal 'yoking' of the cerebral hemispheres, in this view of schizophrenia the cognitive activity in one hemisphere proceeds without, or independent from, that in the other hemisphere – giving rise to 'independent selves' which are unlikely to be given such autonomy in normal individuals. According to the homotopic inhibitory model of callosal functions, a decrease in interhemispheric information transfer could occur due to two forms of pathology: (i) morphological-neurotransmitter abnormalities of the corpus callosum itself – presumably a congenital condition, or (ii) asymmetries of hemispheric arousal – presumably a functional 'acquired' condition. Poor interhemispheric transfer due to asymmetrical (non-homotopic) connections or impaired impulse transmission would lead to impaired topographical transfer of information from hemisphere to hemisphere (regardless of whether it was excitatory or inhibitory). Somewhat less obvious, asymmetrical hemispheric arousal would also impair information transfer – but only if the transfer were inhibitory. That is, if callosal communication normally occurs by means of topographical inhibition between subcortically aroused bilateral 'foci of attention,' then the unilateral attenuation of arousal effects would prevent information transfer – despite the normality of the corpus callosum itself and the cerebral cortex of both hemispheres. In other words, an attentional (primarily subcortical) asymmetry could result in impaired interhemispheric communication. In contrast, if an excitatory mechanism of callosal communication is the normal condition, subcortical mechanisms would be less important in determining the flow of information between the cerebral hemispheres.

The evidence supporting the 'partial deconnection' view of schizophrenia is yet insufficient to draw firm conclusions (Dimond, 1979b); but it is of interest that current research in schizophrenia brings together precisely these two themes – the vertical (or 'arousal') and the horizontal (or 'lateral specializations') aspects of brain function (see Flor-Henry, 1983, and Claridge and Broks, 1984, for further discussion). Clear indications of asymmetric arousal in psychopathological states, including schizophrenia, mania and depression, have been demonstrated in several psychophysiological studies (see Flor-Henry, 1983, and Gruzelier and Flor-Henry, 1979), but possible connections with deficits of interhemispheric communication remain unproven.

The nature of cellular and atomic pathology is only of peripheral interest in the present context, but the relevant information is outlined in table 7.6 It is particularly interesting that at each of these three fundamental levels, the systemic pathology occurring with 'excessive influences' of the external, rather than the internal, control element is the more malignant form of pathology. Excesses of the internal control element also lead to characteristic pathological instabilities of the system, but not to conditions which are as apt to disrupt the system itself. In a word, external control pathology leads to explosive, destructive malignancy, whereas internal control pathology leads to a benign condition of stagnancy.

Table 7.6 The pathology of control in natural systems

System	Externally oriented control element	Internally oriented control element	Excess or hyperactivity of:	
			External element	Internal element
Atom	Proton	Neutron	Nuclear radioactivity (alpha-decay, $beta^+$-decay, fission)	Nuclear radioactivity $beta^-$-decay)
Cell	RNA	DNA	Malignant neoplastic growth (RNA-virus induced)	Benign neoplastic growth (DNA-virus induced)
Human organism	Left hemisphere	Right hemisphere	Schizophrenia	Depression

Summary

The central dogmas of molecular biology and atomic physics are concerned with more than nuclear functions. The genetic code explains not only the interactions of the nucleic acids, but also the mechanism of translation of nucleic acid information into protein form. Indeed the latter half of that central dogma is the more complex half, but it followed logically and chronologically from an understanding of the storage and transmission of information by the nucleic acids (although the reverse was true in atomic physics!).

In atomic physics the interaction of the nucleons is the central topic underlying all aspects of nuclear energy, whereas the proton–electron interaction might justifiably be labeled the essence of chemistry – for the electrostatic interaction between protons and electrons determines the binding forces and distances of the atoms in molecular, ionic or crystalline structures and therefore their chemical reactivity.

In this light it is apparent that the present hypothesis concerning the communication between the cerebral hemispheres is but one part of a complete 'central dogma' for psychology, but it does point to a whole new variety of brain dynamics. Specifically, inhibitory topographical mapping is the second of only *two* possible mechanisms by which spatially encoded neural information can be transmitted to another region of the brain. Contrary to first expectations, inhibition does *not* mean an absence of information in the inhibited region, provided that the effects of surround inhibition (and its inhibition) are also considered.

Previous ideas concerning the brain code have been based exclusively upon excitatory interactions (albeit, making use of inhibitory effects to 'sharpen' the excitatory image). Although little in addition to hopeful speculation is to be found concerning brain code mechanisms beyond the stage of topographical mapping, there can be no doubt that such excitatory mapping is the essence of at least one major part of the brain code. The central remaining question is: 'How does the brain proceed subsequent to its successful construction of topographical sensory maps?' As Phillips *et al.* (1984) exclaim, 'Most of us would like to think the cortex does more than simply disseminate information,' but it would seem that nothing beyond the 'dissemination' of sensory maps is now known.

The obvious direction in which to proceed theoretically in terms of excitatory mapping is to consider more complex mapping among different modalities and submodalities. Sensations of heat and cold, touch, pain and pressure could each separately be mapped with colors, textures, moving edges, high and low auditory frequencies, etc. – but even all such combinations do not lead us beyond the intrinsic limitations of excitatory sensory maps. That is, combinations of sensory stimuli do not lead to concepts; there is no implicit mechanism for producing generalizations based upon specific stimuli. And here, more than anywhere else, lies the fundamental limitations of the computer/ brain analogy. Computers are good at *deduction*: taking the information in memory and wringing every possible combination and permutation out of it. As a consequence, models of human cognition which are based upon deductive processes can readily be implemented within computer programs, and quickly out-perform their human creators. But inductive reasoning has remained a virtual impossibility because the computer has no way of knowing when to conclude that a number of examples of a structure, function or phenomenon indicates a general law, or to know which features of a given phenomenon are representative of general principles and which are peculiar to the observed phenomenon.

It would be wrong to belittle the importance of excitatory topo-graphical mapping within the complete brain code (or deductive thought processes in both man and machine), but map-making appears to be only one aspect of *intra*hemispheric processing. Even complex multimodal excitatory maps are merely the higher end of sensory mapping – important, but leaving the neuronal computer no more capable of generalization and induction than any memory-storage device. Insofar as topographical inhibition provides such a mechanism, it may be the case that the excitatory mechanisms are the principal *intra*hemispheric means for information storage, and inhibitory mechanisms are the principal *inter*hemispheric means for information analysis and manipulation.

Returning to the 'vertical' and 'horizontal' conceptions of the central nervous system, it is of interest that we are led to the mirror-image negative hypothesis only when both dimensions are considered together. Without a simultaneous, bilaterally effective arousal mechanism, callosal inhibition could result in only a quantitative asymmetry of cortical activity which physiological studies have not detected. While interhemispheric inhibition seems essential for explaining much of the laterality literature, only topographical inhibition produces complementary informational content in the cerebral hemispheres, as distinct from separate specializations. We thereby avoid the *prima facie* absurdity that the largest nerve tract in the human brain and the most rapidly evolving tract in phylogeny works only to suppress its neighbor, conveying no information between the hemispheres! We are also not left with the enigma of largely duplicated neural information in the two cerebral hemispheres – as the excitatory model implies.

The deciphered codes of atomic physics and cellular biology are each based upon three fundamental structural elements and their functional relationships. It has been argued that the fundamentals of the 'brain code' can be understood in terms of an isomorphic three-element system with again a small number of important functional relationships.

The 'external' control element of the mammalian brain is that cerebral hemisphere which, for any given task, controls the activity of peripheral musculature to exert desired effects on the external world. In man the externally oriented hemisphere is most frequently the left hemisphere; it is 'dominant' for most speech and skilled manual activities and it remains 'dominant' over the individual's entire lifetime. The 'nondominant' hemisphere has the important 'stability' function of maintaining the cognitive context within which left hemispheric speech comprehension and generation occurs. In other mammalian species, a 'dominant' hemisphere is normally found for individual complex tasks – but it is a 'dominance' which is consistent over time only for the given task.

The nature of 'nondominant' hemisphere functions in animals is less certain – but to the degree that animal brains have homotopic commissural connections between the left and right hemispheres, bilateral cortical information can take the form of either excitatory mirror-images or inhibitory mirror-image 'negatives' of one another. The former implies an approximate duplication of information and the latter implies its transformation into a 'complementary' form.

The 'contextual' role of the right hemisphere in human beings (reviewed in chapter 4) suggests that an inhibitory corpus callosum could be the mechanism through which important *cognitive* asymmetries are generated, but the lack of explicit demonstration of such topographical mapping prevents firm conclusions concerning the actual mechanisms. If the corpus callosum is inhibitory in the sense developed in chapters 3 and 4, then there is a striking isomorphism in terms of structure, function and information flow among the atom, cell and human organism. If the corpus callosum works in a more complex fashion or is not responsible for the 'contextual' role of the right hemisphere, then only structural and functional similarities among these 'control systems' of nature are certain, and questions concerning the mechanisms of information flow remain to be answered.

8

CONCLUSIONS

The evolutionary context

The century following the publication of Darwin's *Origin of Species* (1859) may well be looked upon as 'the era of evolution.' Not only was the diversity of plant and animal organisms placed within a sensible theoretical framework, but also the concepts of gradual change and complexification have become central to our understanding of the physical, biological and social worlds. It is now widely believed that, at a microscopic level, the evolution of the elementary constituents of matter occurred in a few split-seconds following the big-bang origin of the universe. Thereafter further atomic evolution has occurred and continues to occur due to fission and fusion processes which readjust the elementary particles into more stable atomic states. At a macroscopic level, these atomic processes result in the large-scale evolution of stars and planets – and thereby allow for the further evolution of chemical, biological and social entities on the surface of those celestial bodies. Although the time-scale of celestial evolution is so large that such changes do not often affect us directly, nonetheless, both the atomic and celestial aspects of physical evolution are important parts of the modern dynamic view of the universe – arguably ushered in by Darwin and colleagues, if developed by twentieth-century physicists, such as Gamow and Rutherford.

While academic debates concerning the rate and mechanisms of biological evolution continue to be waged, there is little doubt in the scientific community that the biological world is unfolding in a non-deterministic fashion from originally simpler forms into more complex forms. Here, more than elsewhere, the dynamic nature of physical reality has fundamentally revolutionized how the world is perceived. The 'natural order' is not an immutable constant, but a dynamic process – fired by genetic changes and continually evolving due to competition and natural selection. Moreover, although the 'evolution' of social systems requires qualification, it is true that, viewed historically, societies change and usually complexify in response to both internal social factors and external environmental pressures. Again a dynamic, non-deterministic view of social structures (which at least some would prefer to view as static and preordained) has become the established scientific conception of the modern world.

But if the century following the *Origin of Species* can be called 'the era of evolution,' then the era which has followed may well come to be known as 'the era of fitness.' That is to say, accepting that there are processes of 'selection' and weeding out of unstable structures at various levels of natural organization, the era following Darwin's may eventually be considered as the age during which the principles of 'fitness' or viable systemic organization have begun to be elucidated. Not only can answers be found to questions about historically *what* has happened, but also some answers to the *how* and *why* of evolution are becoming possible.

Certainly one major *how* of biological evolution, natural selection, has been a major theme of Darwin's revolution from the outset, but it is one thing to say that the fit survive and another to define what is meant by fitness. Since before Darwin, biologists have noted that a furry mantle or hoofed feet or warm blood, etc., could be advantageous in certain environments, but only with the clarity of modern science is it apparent how such individual cases reflect general principles of viable systemic organization. Herein lies the major lessons of cybernetics and general systems theory: although all existing systems which have evolved through physical, biological or social evolution can be studied as successful examples of systems suited to particular environments, more importantly, any such system can be viewed as one which, through specific mechanisms, can maintain a constant internal structure regardless of the vicissitudes of the external world. By studying the internal dynamics of natural systems, the cybernetic era has been able to delve beneath the phenomenological description of evolution into the mechanisms involved.

So, while the broad stroke of Darwin's brush may provide a picture of change and continuing complexification (to the consternation of the creationists), the detailed knowledge of modern biology and cybernetic theory tells, above all else, of the mechanisms for maintaining constancy (to the consternation of advocates of a thermodynamic, random mutation-driven philosophy of life). In abstract terms, this knowledge has been formalized within general systems theory in the jargon of cybernetics and control system homeostasis and, in the real world, applied in (bio-)chemical engineering, computer-regulated manufacturing processes and robot systems. As far apart as the worlds of evolutionary theory and automated factories may seem, a conceptual link lies in the importance of internal communications for maintaining the coordinated self-regulation of a wide variety of 'systems' over extended periods of time.

While the subcomponents and specific mechanisms of natural and artificial systems may change, fundamental principles of systemic organization remain unaltered. Their elucidation has led and will undoubtedly continue to lead to both a greater understanding of the natural world and more appropriate control over it. This is particularly evident in terms of atomic physics and cellular biology. The atomic and genetic codes which modern science has elegantly deciphered provide the detailed mechanisms through which the atomic and cellular systems maintain long-term stability – maintaining characteristic features in the face of a potentially disruptive environment – and simultaneously allowing for gradual changes which do not destroy the system as a functional whole. In the biological world there is the stabilizing DNA – wrapped around itself in a relatively inert double helix, wound into chromosomes and protected by the nuclear membrane – and the hard-working RNA – taking the genetic information for usage in the cellular cytoplasm in order to make changes in its immediate and extracellular biochemical environment. Moreover, there are known mechanisms of change – commonly labelled with the catch-all rubric 'mutation,' but including a variety of complex, non-random means for altering, amplifying and recombining the cell's genetic structure either by acting directly on DNA or going through an RNA intermediary. In the atomic world constancy is achieved, above all else, by means of the neutron's contribution to nuclear structure – binding strongly to all intranuclear nucleons, while 'mutations' of the atomic system are brought about either by external insult to the nucleus or through the intranuclear repulsive effects of local protons.

Some details of the mechanisms of change and constancy in the brain have become known, but the elegance and clarity found in the atomic and cellular 'central dogmas' have not yet been achieved. On the one hand, some of the initial stages of learning, such as the brain mechanisms of perception, are well understood and some of the principles of efferent motor activity are known, but the physiology involved in the processing of percepts into short-term or long-term memory remains problematical:

> Concepts of mapping and representation of visual space are largely derived from electrophysiological studies in which the receptive fields of single cells or groups of cells are plotted. Is this approach suitable when seeking to understand the higher functions of the cerebral cortex? (Phillips et al., 1984).

The honest answer is that no one knows but, in practical terms, the assumed answer is an emphatic 'Yes' – which allows the techniques of sensory physiology to be used as the problems under study become more abstract and admittedly distant from the problems of raw sensation. While the detailed mechanisms of sensation become increasingly well understood, there is no certainty that the rich harvest of sensory physiology will ever result in a coherent central dogma for cognitive psychology.

The way forward for the brain sciences is not entirely clear, but at least some of the problems in defining a psychological central dogma may come simply from a failure to define the level at which a dogma is needed. For better or worse, academic 'psychology' embraces topics from the molecules involved in synaptic transmission to the organizational dynamics of business corporations. So when psychologists discuss 'the brain code,' they often mean very different things – depending largely upon individual research interests. Some will be excited solely by the transformation of light stimuli into visual images – and the phrase 'brain code' will be used to mean phenomena within the visual system up to but not including association cortex. Some will be interested in the translation of sounds into phonetic units in auditory cortex and meaningful symbols somewhere beyond. Others will be interested in the transformation of plans – somehow formulated in frontal cortex – into motor activity. Still braver souls will be concerned with the problem of reading or writing in response to auditory dictation or the neural correlates of creativity. It is noteworthy, however, that whether essentially sensory, motor or associative, each of these issues can be dealt with conceptually within a *single* hemisphere (figure 8.1). From synaptic transmission to high-level polymodal associations, the *bilaterality* of nervous systems has usually been an irrelevancy or simply a convenient control configuration (since each animal provides an intact hemisphere as an internal control on the effects of contralateral meddling).

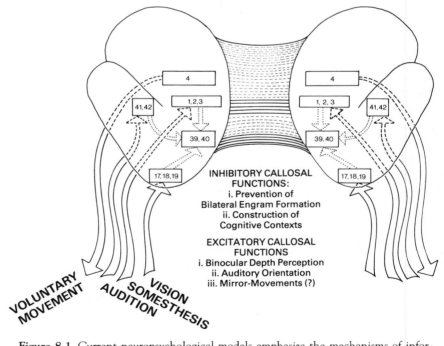

Figure 8.1 Current neuropsychological models emphasize the mechanisms of information transfer to and from a single, usually the left, hemisphere. The significance of corticocortical connections and particularly callosal functions remain obscure.

It is of course recognized by all that in real brains virtually any brain phenomenon involves massive and continual interhemispheric effects, but proposed information-processing routes usually involve structures, all of which are located within only one hemisphere or which work autonomously in parallel in the two hemispheres. Over the past two decades, parallel routes within the right hemisphere have attracted attention, but again the emphasis has been on a self-contained right hemisphere, rather than on left–right interactions. As a research program this emphasis on the vertical structure of the brain has proven to be a valid starting-point, but it must be recognized as the convenient fiction which it is. At some stage, it will become necessary to tackle the problem of interhemispheric communication.

It is noteworthy that, in research on visual perception, the second stage has recently been reached. First, the fundamental mechanisms of vision were elucidated without concern for interhemispheric effects and (while further progress in the understanding of the 'vertical' structure of vision continues) only subsequently has it been necessary or even possible to consider interhemispheric processes for an understanding of binocular vision and depth perception.

The preceding seven chapters might be viewed as a lengthy statement on the importance of interhemispheric effects and a declaration that the time may now have been reached for a shift in emphasis toward the horizontal, corticocortical aspects of brain function. In other words, insofar as important mechanisms of communication may be revealed by studying how the two cerebral hemispheres interact, the laterality issue may be a more profound topic than most 'left self, right self' popularizations would suggest. Although two autonomous 'brains' may be a more realistic view than a single 'dominant' brain, two interacting 'brains' is more realistic yet! If in fact mechanisms of interhemispheric communication constitute a fundamental *class* of brain dynamics, then it may well be that, in the search for the fundamental rules of the brain code, in general brain scientists will be taking an unnecessarily difficult route, if interhemispheric processes are set aside for later study.

Be that as it may, it is unquestionably the case that, today amidst many technical and conceptual achievements, discussion of candidate universal mechanisms involved in the brain code has become increasingly rare. Although there seems to be some agreement that a common 'cortical language' is likely, few are intrepid enough to offer suggestions concerning the ground rules which might apply equally well, for example, to auditory cortex and motor cortex (see the historical overview by Phillips et al., 1984). The ground rules of *neuronal* functioning have in fact been known for several decades and have led to speculation concerning a few general classes of possible 'brain codes' – none of which has yet proven itself as the fundamental cornerstone of brain functioning.

Abeles (1982) has identified three classes of 'brain code:' (i) the mass action hypothesis, (ii) the dedicated line hypothesis and (iii) Abeles's own 'synchronous firing chain' hypothesis. The mass action hypothesis postulates that the activity of a large number of neurons is involved in any sensory or motor event – with no uniquely competent specialized modules. The degree of neural damage is therefore predicted and, roughly speaking, found to correlate with the degree of behavioral deficit – quite aside from the location of the brain damage. The 'holographic' theory of Pribram is a modern version of 'mass action.' The dedicated line hypothesis is usually characterized (by opponents) as the grandmother cell theory, since it demands separate neurons for each and every object and phenomenon in the external world (including your grandmother). Abeles's synchronous firing chain hypothesis was devised to avoid the apparent lack of specificity in the mass action hypothesis and the excessive specificity required in the dedicated line theory. He maintains that through repeated usage and a mechanism of positive feedback, a set of neurons which is originally a random collection becomes specialized for a given task. Eventually a unique set of neurons fires in synchrony in response to specified stimuli – approaching the specificity of the dedicated line hypothesis, but starting from the non-specificity of the mass action hypothesis.

In contrast, Uttal (1978) has identified eight potential factors involved in 'the neural language' – each of which may be an important part of the three mechanisms proposed by Abeles. They include: (i) place (the location within the nervous system which is activated by an incoming signal), (ii) number of activated units, (iii) the neural event amplitude and (iv) the temporal pattern. The temporal pattern itself can be broken into: (v) graded potential time functions (the shape of the neural response), (vi) frequency of firing, (vii) micro- and macro-fluctuations in the frequency pattern and (viii) derived statistical measures (auto- and cross-correlations and entropy measures).

Empirically the known 'codes' of the brain cover only much smaller segments of what a complete brain code must accomplish. What is perhaps most striking about the candidate codes of Abeles and Uttal is that they are pitched at such different levels. Each of Abeles's 'codes' encompasses sensation, cognition and motor output, whereas Uttal's 'codes' are elementary neuronal mechanisms which may be at work anywhere in the nervous system. The empirical findings on the sensory and motor cortical maps, on the other hand, are the phenomenological facts known at the early sensory and late motor stages of nervous processing in the brain code, but clearly represent only a momentary slice of time through any one of Abeles's start-to-finish models, and may occur through the workings of any or all of Uttal's neuron codes!

Are we therefore at a conceptual impasse, where we are simply incapable of comprehending the implications of such a large number of possibilities? Judging from the popularity of the phrase that 'the human brain may not be capable of comprehending itself,' it would appear that many despair of the possibility of a 'brain code,' but I am not convinced that success is far away. Arguably our main task at this time is simply to define what needs to be done and, implicitly, what cannot now be done.

In analogy with research in molecular biology, it is easy to see with the aid of hindsight that the nucleotide sequence which codes for, say, a specific membrane protein could not have been deduced in the mid-1950s directly from even a complete understanding of DNA stereochemistry. Even knowing that genes are sequences of specific nucleotides, the mechanisms for translating those sequences into amino acid chains required elucidation before anything concrete could be said about the relationship between a particular genotype and a particular phenotype.

To be sure, given a few decades of research, the problems of determining the DNA sequences of specific proteins (and still trickier problems reminiscent of the 'brain comprehending itself,' such as determining the DNA sequence for a protein that checks and repairs DNA sequences!) have been solved. But the starting-point – now nearly forgotten amidst the various developments which have allowed for genetic engineering – was a radically simplistic idea concerning the stereochemical complementarity of the nucleotide bases. Could the neurosciences be in a comparable post-DNA/pre-biotechnology stage of development, without having realized that the first few major hurdles have already been crossed?

Although we do not know all of the spatial and temporal elements of the neuron code, we do know the fundamentals of the spatial aspects of the sensory and motor cortical maps. Together with the fact that the neuronal configuration of the adult brain is not malleable (in the sense of being able to establish and reestablish anatomical connectivity rapidly) and neurons can only excite or inhibit one another, it is most likely that excitatory topographical mapping – from literal mapping of the external world to gradually more abstract polymodal mapping – is the most fundamental *informational* process of the brain code. In

Table 8.1 A summary of possible mechanisms of corticocortical communication

	Net excitatory effects	Net inhibitory effects
The spatial configuration of the tracts is informational	Topographical excitatory mapping – 'mirror-image' positives	Topographical inhibitory mapping – 'mirror-image' negatives
The spatial configuration of the tracts is non-informational	Diffuse excitatory arousal	Diffuse inhibitory de-arousal

addition to the projection and distorted reprojection of those sensory maps, inhibitory mapping may allow for the production of novel emphasis of elements within such maps.

The second 'dimension' of corticocortical communication involves more diffuse effects. When one region (modality, submodality, etc.) is active, other regions can, as a consequence, also become activated or contrarily become deactivated. As shown in table 8.1 these four categories of cortical communication are identical to the four current hypotheses concerning callosal function (see table 3.1). Although interhemispheric communication is *atypical* in being largely the communication between two anatomically similar structures and although the corpus callosum is *atypical* in being an exposed and seemingly unitary structure, callosal mechanisms may be representative of how, in general, the brain communicates with itself.

Implications for artificial intelligence

One of the central problems in achieving computer systems which can act in intelligent ways is to teach computers to function within the appropriate context of ongoing linguistic communication. For normal people this ability seems trivial. Using a vast storehouse of memories concerning things which actually have happened, we have definite expectations about what is likely to happen or what people are likely to say. Although there seems to be no limit to the amount of information which ultimately can be stored in computers, a major difficulty in producing truly intelligent computers comes in generating reasonable expectations and in retrieving the appropriate information without going through the entire memory store. A typical example of a sentence which today's computers would spend too much time and effort on is:

> He punched him in the nose and he fell over backwards, but he did not apologize to him.

This is perhaps not a very well-constructed sentence but, for normal brains, only a moment's *reflection* is required to sort out the likely chain of events from among a number of bizarre possibilities. We are not normally led astray by the inherent ambiguity in such sentences because we do not wade through a linear series of all possible meanings looking for the probable meaning. Somehow we seem to process all of the possibilities and only one or possibly a few stand out as likely.

The topic of how such 'disambiguation' can be achieved in computers is only one part of research on computer intelligence, but it is representative of the kinds of problems which are being encountered in research on artificial intelligence. Basically computers appear to be capable of virtually any kind of processing which people are capable of specifying – but the machines have problems in knowing where to start, when to quit and how to avoid the entire realm of 'obvious' irrelevancies. It is simply not feasible to plod through every logical possibility; in order for machines to become 'intelligent' they require means for putting their massive data-processing capabilities within appropriate contexts.

It is of interest, therefore, to consider how the human brain accomplishes this – in order to see what the brain sciences might suggest to the computer sciences. As discussed in chapter 4 psychological research on brain-damaged patients has led to a characterization of the left hemisphere as being somewhat like a literal, plodding 'language machine' – linguistically capable, but often 'missing the point' (Gardner *et al.*, 1983). Superficially the right-hemisphere-damaged patient appears to be normally 'intelligent,' but tends not to understand metaphors or jokes, fails to express the usual emotions which accompany the proper understanding of language, and cannot distinguish between likely and non-sequitur endings to short narratives. Would the hard-headed AI researcher consider such patients to be 'intelligent'? Probably not – simply because they lack precisely the contextual, framework-building capabilities which transform 'data-processing' into 'insight.'

If the left and right cerebral hemispheres are in fact responsible for respectively the literal and contextual understanding of language, then two obvious implications for artifical intelligence are immediately apparent. The first is simply that disambiguation and context-building is of such major importance and so inherently complex that, in effect, an entire hemisphere of the brain is used for these functions. While one hemisphere is involved in the phonetic encoding and decoding of language, as well as the syntactic parsing and first-order denotative decoding which is required for the literal understanding of linguistic messages, the other hemisphere is involved in disambiguation and higher-order semantic decoding. In this view, contextual disambiguation is not one of several crucial steps in the linear decoding of language, it is *the* major parallel process which is undertaken simultaneously with the denotative language functions studied in classical linguistics.

A second and more interesting implication of such a neural structure lies in the functional relationship between *two roughly equivalent* 'processors' which are bound together and forced to work in unison due to massive interconnections. Although the necessity of *multi*processors and simultaneously occurring number-crunching among *many* parallel devices is real enough in various realms of computing, it may be that the context problem should be approached in terms of interacting *dual* processors – where one processor is involved directly in the literal aspects of language decoding (primarily syntactical ordering and literal semantic decoding), and the other is involved in using each element of language to generate an overall, coherent, if less precise, semantic framework.

So, when the computer is told, for example, that 'George threw a ball,' it will know immediately whether this refers to a sphere propelled

215

through the air or a dance held for charity. The ambiguity will be resolved from the sum total of previously understood contextual signs (references to the back yard and a sore arm, on the one hand, or dancing, tuxedos and champagne, on the other) and their known relations with 'ball' in the established semantic network, rather than from a grinding analysis of all logical possibilities. Mellish's (1985) concept of ongoing semantic processing, where disambiguation runs in parallel with, rather than following after syntactical processing, is a good example of how computers can be persuaded to function in such psychologically realistic ways.

The topic of dual processors is not in fact new to computing. A common configuration is the so-called master–slave relationship between two identical processors. Here the master processor will relegate many of the chores involved in external communication to the slave. So having achieved, for example, a numerical result, the master processor will display it on the screen or print it on the printer by way of the slave processor. A rough similarity with the cerebral hemispheres might be perceived here (with the left hemisphere being the slave!), but it is not a profound similarity since, in computers, there does not occur truly parallel and complementary processing in such coprocessors. In the conventional master–slave configuration, there is effectively only one central processor, with a second processor used as a part of the effector apparatus.

From the perspective of artificial intelligence, and specifically the problem of disambiguation, the qualitative problem of how *complementary coprocessing* can be achieved for simultaneous literal and contextual understanding would appear to be a more important issue than the quantitative increases in computational speed promised by *multi*parallel processors. To discover means through which parallel semantic nets might be made to respond to stimuli in complementary ways would be to contribute to the design of intelligent computers and perhaps to shed more light on the detailed mechanisms of how living brains achieve this.

Final remarks

Several comprehensive reviews of cortical processing have recently been published (e.g. Merzenich and Kaas, 1980) – with emphasis on the fundamental nature of cortical *topographical* representations. Recognition of the importance of inhibitory processes throughout the nervous system has been growing steadily for several decades – both in terms of the physiology of perception (contrast enhancement, etc.) and in terms of computer simulation of brain activities. The inhibitory nature of normal callosal activity has also received considerable attention over the last ten years, but the theoretical possibility of *inhibitory topographical mapping* has not previously been explored – primarily, I believe, because of the failure to appreciate the fundamental *bilaterality* of brainstem arousal effects. In a word, while the duality of the human nervous system has been 'rediscovered' (in 'two brain' theory), the simultaneity of the hemispheric 'coprocessors' has not been appreciated. Only within the context of simultaneous *bilateral arousal* do inhibitory processes become of interest. Without *bilateral* processing, inhibitory effects can lead only to ideas about global hemispheric 'suppression' and to unwarranted emphasis on disparate and sometimes contradictory right-hemispheric 'talents' and left-hemispheric 'talents,' but not to complementary interactions. Perhaps it can be said that most of the dead-ends which 'two brain' theory has lured us into have now been sufficiently explored and abandoned, and attention can shift to the nature of the possible interactions of the two hemispheres.

The integrationist perspective on hemisphere functions has been emphasized by Gazzaniga and Kinsbourne, among others, and the attentional mechanisms of the brainstem have been resurrected after several decades by Crick. Together with recent work of Gardner, Gainotti and others on the importance of the high-level cognitive capabilities of the right hemisphere and on the interaction between literal and contextual understanding in artificial intelligence (e.g. Mellish), these core issues may yet give psychology its long-awaited 'central dogma.'

Appendix 1
MAPS OF THE CEREBRAL CORTEX

In chapter 2 the construction of a two-dimensional cortical map was outlined to provide a framework for studying the spatial transformations of cortical information. In this appendix further details of the maps are provided. The merits of the two-dimensional view of the cortex lie mainly in that they depict the brain in a simplified manner which highlights its capacity for two-dimensional representations of the external world. For some perhaps, no more needs to be said than simply that the cortex takes a complex sensory field and represents it in two dimensions, but the maps drive the point home and I believe force us to conceptualize cortical activity in a useful and realistic way.

The size of the various regions in the figures of this appendix are drawn in accordance with the areal values obtained by Henneberg (1910), who measured the surface areas of the entire cerebral cortex of seven normal human cerebral hemispheres (four European Caucasians, one Hottentot, one Javan and one Herero). Unfortunately he did not study differences between the hemispheres from each specimen, but a number of his findings are of interest. The frontal lobes from the seven brains constituted 33–8 percent of the total cortical surface and the limbic lobe constituted 7–11 percent. The major lobes and lobules are shown in figure A1.1 and the prominent gyri and sulci are depicted in figure A1.2.

Anatomical work done many decades ago must of course be viewed with caution. There are, however, two reasons for placing some trust in the areal values which Henneberg reported in 1910. Most importantly the mean surface area is within 5 percent of the values reported recently by Elias and Schwartz (1969), who used a presumably more precise stereological method. Secondly, if we were to be particularly unfriendly to Henneberg and suspect that his comparative measures of brain sizes were motivated by ethnological biases concerning the superiority of west European man, we would expect to find indication of his biases in the reported comparisons among the races. In fact the mean surface areas which he reports were similar among his specimens with notably the largest frontal lobes found in the Hottentot brain. As noted in chapter 2 there is also good agreement with other reported measures in terms of surface areas of the major lobes and in terms of the total surface area of the brain. The relative and absolute measures therefore appear to be as good as any available.

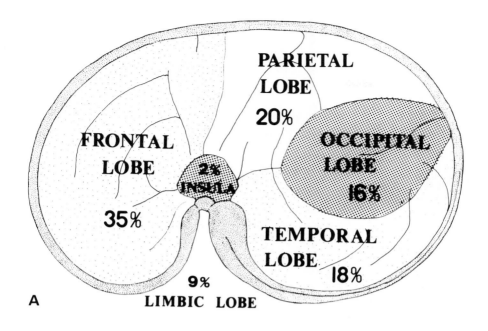

A

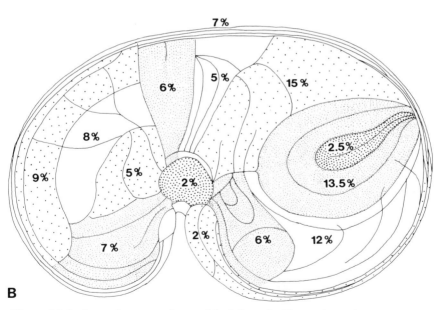

B

Figure A1.1 A two-dimensional map of the left cerebral hemisphere of man. (A) The major lobes. (B) The areas of various lobules. Percentages indicate the average values obtained by Henneberg (1910), with the addition of the 2.5% value for visual striate cortex from von Economo (1929). Note the central location of the insular cortex and its contiguity with the limbic system.

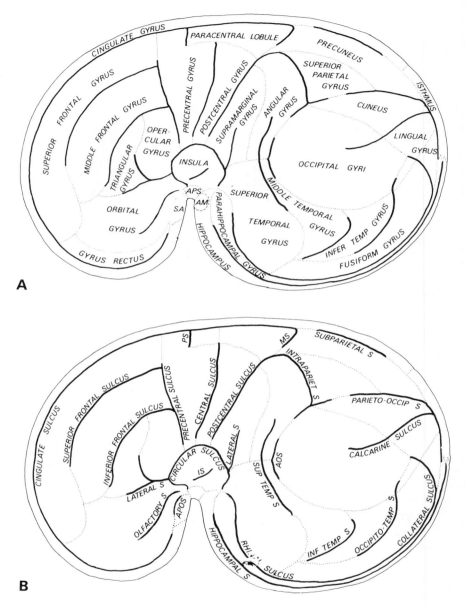

Figure A1.2 The relative positions of the major gyri (A) and sulci (B). Since there is some discrepancy in the commonly used terminology, the following definitions should be noted. The inferior parietal gyrus is comprised of the supramarginal and angular gyri. Both the lingual gyrus (i.e. the medial occipito-temporal gyrus) and the fusiform gyrus (i.e. the lateral occipito-temporal gyrus) cover regions of both the occipital and temporal lobes. The inferior temporal gyrus is often defined as including the region between the inferior temporal sulcus and the occipito-temporal sulcus (i.e. the inferior temporal gyrus proper) and the fusiform gyrus. However, since such definition entails

Brodmann's areas are shown in figures A1.3 (after Brodmann's original diagrams) and A1.4, which is a comparison of the maps of chapter 2 with a similar map drawn by Denning (1966). Because of the stretching of the cortex to produce such a map, the cingulate region and particularly the isthmal area are not easily identified in relation to major sulci. Areas 13–16 and 48–51 are not clearly denoted in Brodmann's original work, but they are thought to lie either on the insula and anterior perforated substance or on the opercular regions of the frontal, parietal and temporal lobes which overhang the insula (Elliot, 1969).

Note the heavy dashed line in figure A1.4(A) which defines the exposed lateral surface of the brain. All regions outside of the dashed line lie on the medial surface of the brain along the interhemispheric fissure or deep within the medio-orbital surface near the brainstem. Note also the location of the frontal, occipital and temporal poles (denoted by large Xs).

The precise boundaries of thalamocortical radiations remain controversial because of differences among species and the inevitable limitations on experimental work on human brains. Delineation of the regions of projection from the various 'association' and 'nonspecific' nuclei is, however, important for understanding brain function. That is insofar as inhibitory or excitatory topographical mapping requires the simultaneous arousal of separate brain regions which are connected by association fibers, information transfer can occur only between regions with the necessary anatomical connections (both corticocortical and subcortical). Sensory relay thalamic nuclei project to well-defined areas of the occipital, temporal and parietal lobes, but the cortical distributions of the nonspecific and associational nuclei via indirect routes are complex and often remain to be confirmed in man. Current findings indicate a map of thalamocortical radiations such as in figure A1.5, but future refinements are likely. As discussed in chapter 3 the importance of the nonspecific input to the neocortex cannot be overemphasized, but it should be noted that the essence of the nonspecific input may lie precisely in its diffuseness and lack of sharp boundaries.

Broca originally chose the phrase 'limbic lobe' to describe the various structures which he saw as surrounding the brainstem, and subsequent comparative neuroanatomy has shown that the cortical portions of what has come to be known as the 'limbic system' were the first structures to emerge for neural processing beyond the brainstem. The

---

calling a portion of the occipital lobe 'temporal,' in the present account the inferior temporal gyrus is limited to the inferior temporal gyrus proper. The inferior frontal gyrus is comprised of the opercular, triangular and orbital gyri, as well as the gyrus rectus.

Key (A): AM, site of the amygdala, the bulk of which is subcortical; APS, anterior perforated substance; SA, septal area. For further details concerning the limbic system, see figures A1.6–A1.8. Key (B): AOS, anterior occipital sulcus; APOS, anterior parolfactory sulcus; IS, insular sulcus; MS, marginal sulcus; PS, paracentral sulcus.

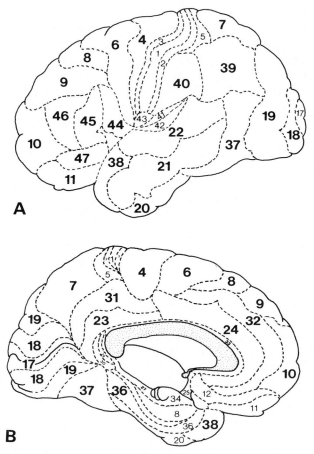

Figure A1.3 Brodmann's cytoarchitectonic map of the cortex. Compare with figure A1.4.

limbic paleocortex was the highest level at which sensory processing could take place – concerned primarily with olfaction, but having connections with all other sensory modalities – thus making it rudimentary 'association cortex.' The limbic lobe is limbic in a second and more interesting sense as well. In the higher vertebrates it is the outer edge of the neocortex – still a major part of the brain in most non-primates, but becoming a minor fringe in the human (and dolphin) brain. Rather than being the final stage of sensory processing, as in reptilian and amphibian brains, it is more accurately characterized as being involved in the descent of neural information from the neocortex. Receiving input from various neocortical areas, the limbic lobe as a whole can be viewed as the second highest neural station in autonomic and neurosecretory motor functions which are ultimately under neocortical control.

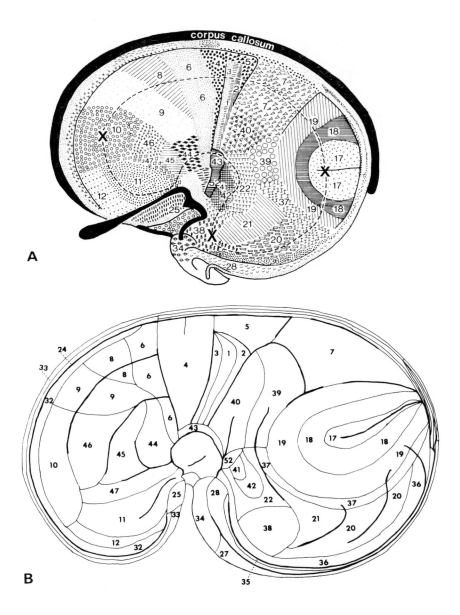

Figure A1.4 Brodmann's areas as represented on two maps of the cortex. (A) Denning's (1966) map. (B) A comparable map undergoing slightly different distortions. Although the relative areas of the lobes are as indicated by Henneberg (1910), the dimensions of Brodmann's areas are only approximate.

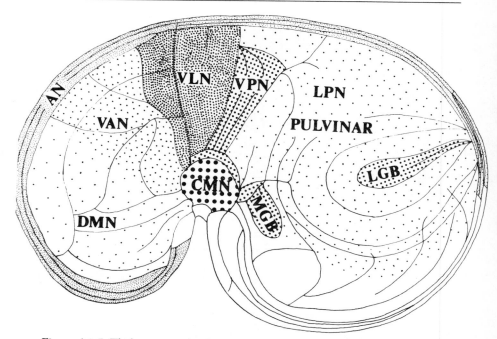

Figure A1.5 Thalamocortical radiations. Note that much of the temporal lobe does not receive thalamic input – roughly the same regions which receive commissural fibers via the anterior commissure rather than the corpus callosum. There is greater specificity of radiations from the various anterior nuclei (AN) of the thalamus to areas within the limbic system than indicated in the figure (see Angevine *et al.*, 1962). Projections from the thalamic centromedian nucleus (CMN) to the insula have been reported but are controversial. Key: (thalamic nuclei): DMN, dorsomedial nucleus; LDN, lateral dorsal nucleus; LGB, lateral geniculate body; LPN, lateral posterior nucleus; MGB, medial geniculate body; VAN, ventral anterior nucleus; VLN, ventral lateral nucleus; VPN, ventral posterior nucleus.

The 'border' nature of the limbic lobe relative to the neocortex can be readily appreciated in the two-dimensional maps of the cortex, where it appears as a narrow border around the neocortical surface. Although relatively small in areal extent, it is contiguous with large portions of all other lobes except the occipital lobe, with which it makes contact only where the calcarine sulcus approaches the isthmus. The fact that the limbic system is also contiguous with brainstem structures is perhaps more clearly evident from White's (1965) schematization, shown in figure A1.6(A). White depicts the limbic lobe as a flattened surface surrounding the foramen of Monro – the opening through which cerebrospinal fluid flows from the midline third ventricle into each of the lateral ventricles. Connections with the brainstem in this depiction would be along the circumference of the foramen of Monro and emerge in the third dimension from the paper. Neocortex would extend out from the outer edge of the limbic lobe and form a neocortical balloon (see figure 2.4).

The anatomy of the limbic lobe is notoriously complex – and made more complex by a contradictory and redundant terminology. Many of the inherent difficulties of limbic structure and function cannot be resolved by any illustration, but the two-dimensional approach does emphasize certain important features of the limbic system which might otherwise be obscure.

Figure A1.6(B) is an enlargement of the central portion of the limbic lobe as depicted in figures A1.1 through A1.5. It illustrates the fact that the principal limbic structures – the hippocampus, amygdala and septal area – are nearly contiguous and feed directly into the hypothalamus. This fact is less evident in usual depictions of the limbic system (see figure A1.7). Nauta and Haymaker (1969) note that

> the hypothalamus is broadly continuous with surrounding grey matter, from which it can be delineated only with difficulty and in some locations only by invoking purely arbitrary topographic criteria. These tissue continuities need to be emphasized, for they express not only topographic relationships but also functional associations. [Surrounding limbic structures can] thus be viewed as intermediaries in the functional associations of the hypothalamus with the rest of the brain.

A similar point is made by Swanson (1983), who has drawn a flattened map of the cortex of the rat (figure A1.8). Although the relative sizes of the cortical areas in the rat brain are different from those in the human brain, the structural similarities are evident – with the limbic lobe appearing as a major part of the cortex comparable to the frontal lobe of man. In the rat brain the hippocampal formation serves as a large polymodal or supramodal association area; only a narrow strip of neocortical association cortex is to be found.

Finally figure A1.9 depicts two versions of cerebral localization – both of which are speculative. Penfield's (1959) depiction of localization is of interest because of its emphasis on higher cerebral functions. Brain stimulation with a mild electric current in awake patients suggests an 'ideational' role of the parietal lobe, but it is evident that the labels on association cortical areas are psychological in nature, whereas those elsewhere are physiological. The link between the two remains uncertain, and cries of 'Phrenology!' will continue to echo in the halls of academia until the translation rules between the two realms are found!

Hrbek's (1976) depiction of cortical function is of interest for its strong emphasis on strictly sensory and motor functions. He denies the reality of even the language areas as 'higher cognitive' regions, and has attempted to view all of brain function solely in terms of input and output without any of the 'idealist's' notions of abstract cognition. Whether or not we can accept Hrbek's extreme position, it does have

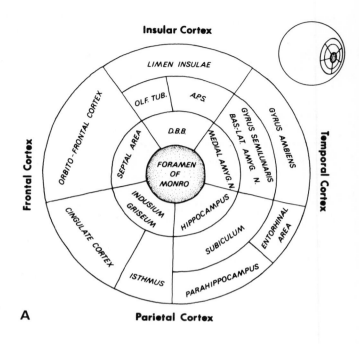

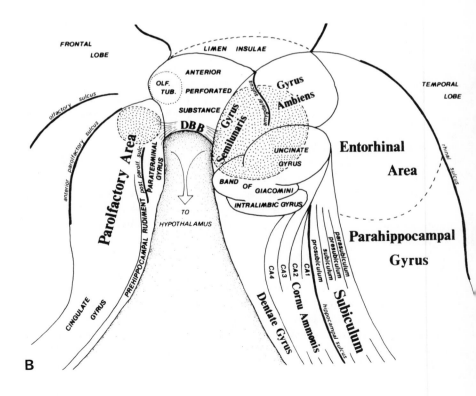

A

B

Figure A1.6 (left) Maps of the limbic lobe. A shows the limbic lobe as viewed from within the third ventricle (modified from White, 1965). White's limbic map would fit on to an inflated left hemisphere as shown in the upper right. B shows an enlargement of the central portion of the limbic lobe in the two-dimensional maps of this appendix. Key: stipled area on left, subcortical location of the nucleus accumbens septi; stipled area on right, subcortical location of the amygdalar complex; DBB, diagonal band of Broca; OLF. TUB., olfactory tubercle.

For those interested in limbic anatomy, the following definitions should be noted. The parolfactory area is synonomous with the septal area, but 'the septum' usually refers to nuclei located within the paraterminal gyrus. The paraterminal gyrus together with the prehippocampal rudiment forms the so-called subcallosal gyrus, which is connected with the hippocampus via the longitudinal striae. Various terms are in use to describe the subdivisions of the limbic system, some of which are noted in the figure. In addition the 'uncus' normally refers to the uncinate gyrus, band of Giacomini and intralimbic gyrus. The 'piriform lobe' includes the entire rostral end of the hippocampal region, i.e. the gyrus ambiens, gyrus semilunaris, uncus and entorhinal area, but excluding the hippocampus. The so-called hippocampal gyrus includes the subiculum, cornu Ammonis and dentate gyrus, but the hippocampus proper is comprised of only the cornu Ammonis and the dentate gyrus. Since, however, there is a gradual transition from hippocampal three-layered cortex to parahippocampal six-layered cortex, this is a matter of fairly arbitrary definition only.

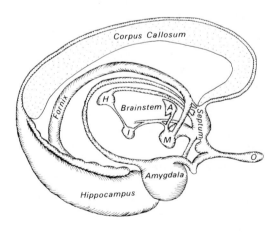

Figure A1.7 MacLean's depiction of the limbic system – anatomically a more realistic drawing than the flattened maps, but one which defies understanding! Key: A, anterior thalamic nuclei; H, habenular nucleus; I, interpeduncular nucleus; M, mammillary body; O, olfactory bulb.

227

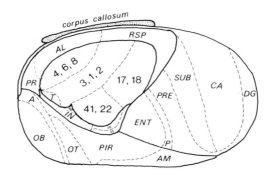

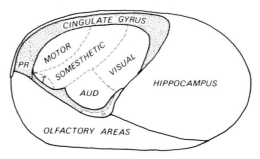

Figure A1.8 A map of the cortex of the left hemisphere of the rat (modified from Swanson, 1983). The architectonically defined areas of the cortex are shown above and the major functional areas below. Compare with figures A1.1 and A1.6. Key: A, anterior olfactory nucleus; AL, anterior limbic area; AM, amygdala; CA, cornu Ammonis; DG, dentate gyrus; ENT, entorhinal area; IN, insula; OB, olfactory bulb; OT, olfactory tubercle; P, parasubiculum; PIR, piriform cortex; PR, prefrontal region; PRE, presubiculum; RSP, retrosplenial area; SUB, subiculum; T, taste area. Regions of polymodal and supramodal association cortex are indicated by the stipling.

interesting implications. Specifically the regions of neocortex which Penfield labels 'ideational,' 'perceptual judgment' and 'elaboration of conscious thought' are seen by Hrbek as being involved in 'proprioceptive' and 'interoceptive-glanduloceptive' input and 'interomotor and secretomotor' output. Instead of abstract cognition, he sees the role of much of 'association' cortex as being involved in 'internal' perceptual and motor processes. Such a theoretical framework might become the basis for a physiologically comprehensible theory of psychosomatic disease which gets away from the abstract constructs of Freudian theory. These possibilities remain unexplored.

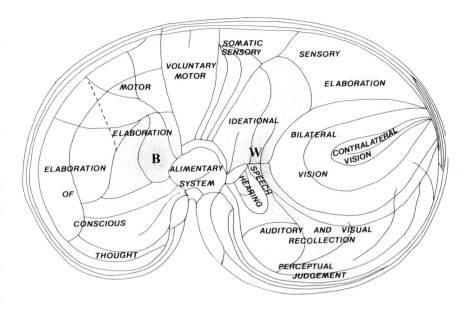

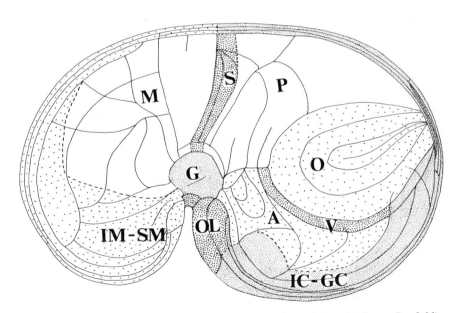

Figure A1.9 Two depictions of cerebral localization. Above are shown Penfield's localized higher functions. B and W indicate the approximate locations of Broca's and Wernicke's areas, respectively. Below is shown Hrbek's localization map, emphasizing only sensory and motor functions. Key: A, auditory; G, gustatory; IC-GC, interoceptive and glanduloceptive; IM-SM, interomotor and secretomotor; M, motor; O, optical; P, proprioceptive; S, somesthetic; V, vestibular.

Appendix 2
COMPUTER SIMULATIONS

Computer simulations of brain activity are useful exercises for at least two reasons. They require that virtually all aspects of the hypothesis under examination be made explicit, and therefore force exploration in directions which might not otherwise be regarded as important. Secondly, although the differences between the real brain and the simulated brain are such that all findings which appear supportive of a given hypothesis must be viewed cautiously, a simulation can indicate certain combinations of assumptions which could not work in the real brain. That is, disproof of certain hypotheses is possible, even if successful simulation will only be demonstration of the capabilities of the computer – not necessarily the living brain. Eventually, when simulations contain sufficiently numerous details concerning neuronal function and sufficiently complex interconnections, stronger conclusions about the real brain may be possible. For the purposes of this appendix, greatly simplified cortical neurons with limited interconnectivity will be used to demonstrate techniques, rather than to draw conclusions.

The two programs which are listed below should prove instructive concerning the possible implications of a topographically organized corpus callosum. Program 1 demonstrates the spatial relationship between patches of cerebral cortex with homotopic callosal connections, and the effects of various kinds of intra- and interhemispheric inhibitory or excitatory effects. Program 2 is a simulation of the temporal aspects of such connectivity, where the adjustable parameters are concerned with the degree of homotopic versus heterotopic connections. Details of a more realistic simulation can be found in Anninos and Cook (1986), but the general principles behind this approach to studying brain function should be apparent from the BASIC programs which follow. The BASIC dialect is MICROSOFT BASIC, but the program should run with only minor changes on any microcomputer with 16K of memory and an 80 column by 25 line screen which can be addressed using commands such as 'LOCATE x, y.'

Simulation 1

First, the underlying assumptions of the simulation concerned with mirror-image projections across the corpus callosum will be presented in

230

a simplified, logical form and then the BASIC programs and typical results will be listed.

It is assumed that: (i) language processes involve the firing of functional units in the cerebral cortex, i.e. 'columns;' (ii) cortical excitation elicits patterns of surround inhibition around activated columns; and (iii) activation also elicits patterns of excitatory or inhibitory effects on the homotopic contralateral cortex. The firing of any given column can be expressed as follows:

$$Z(n) = 1 = TE.CE.\bar{SI}.CI + TE.CE.SI.\bar{CI} + TE.CE.\bar{SI}.\bar{CI}$$
$$= (TE + CE).\bar{SI}.\bar{CI} \qquad (1)$$

where nonspecific thalamocortical excitation is represented by variable TE, corticocortical excitation by variable CE, surround inhibition by variable SI and callosal inhibition by CI.

Since only one hemisphere normally develops the motor control capacities necessary for speech, only one (normally the left) hemisphere will contain appropriate corticocortical inputs which control areas directly involved in language production (variable CE). Furthermore, since speech will normally require conscious attention (presumably requiring non-specific thalamocortical excitation, TE), cortical activity in the left hemisphere can be expressed simply as the third term in Eq. 1

$$Z_{left}(n) = 1 = TE.CE.\bar{SI}.\bar{CI} \qquad (2)$$

resulting in inhibition of the homologous cortical column in the right hemisphere. Due to the largely bilateral nature of subcortical excitation during attention, the subsets of cortical neurons activated via the thalamocortical inputs will be similar in the left and right, but callosal inhibition would prevent the simultaneous firing of homotopic columns. Disregarding the effects of surround inhibition for the moment, it is found that the homologous cortical columns in the left and right hemispheres can be described as

$$Z_{left}(n) = 1\ TE.CE.\bar{CI} \text{ and } Z_{right}(n) = 0 = TE.\bar{CE}.CI \qquad (3)$$

Since surround inhibition is thought to have summatory effects on cortical columns, a given column within the focus of attention will be prevented from firing only when a certain number of neighboring columns are firing simultaneously. Geometrically the densest and therefore most likely two-dimensional configuration of cortical 'cylinders' is hexagonal close-packing (Towe, 1975). If it is assumed that the firing of three or more nearest neighbors in such a configuration is sufficient to inhibit a given column, then the firing of a cortical column in the left hemisphere $[Z_{left}(n) = 1 = TE.CE.\bar{SI}.\bar{CI}]$ will result in one of two forms of contralateral inhibition $[Z_{right}(n) = 0 = TE.CE.\bar{SI}.CI$ or $TE.CE.SI.CI]$ – the former being one of thirty-two possible configurations and the latter one of twenty-two possibilities – depending upon the pattern of surround inhibition acting on the given column in the right hemisphere. In the simulation itself, the implications of any one of the four principal theories of callosal function (table 3.1) can be studied by selecting a callosal hypothesis at the start of the program. A unilateral left hemisphere 'engram' is then constructed by specifying the x- and y-coordinates to be activated in the left hemisphere. The spatial effects of the callosal hypothesis and surround inhibition in both hemispheres are then displayed.

Simulation 2

The second simulation is designed to show how the summed activity in two cortical 'neural nets' can vary depending upon parameters concerning (i) the similarity between the internal connectivity of the two nets, (ii) the percentage of homotopicity of the callosal fibers, and (iii) the percentage of inhibitory and excitatory callosal effects. Unlike simulation one, which is a static 'picture' of two related neural nets, this program is dynamic in the sense that the activity of the two nets is calculated sequentially. Since the sum of active neurons in each state would correspond to the overall electrical activity of the net (as measured somewhere above the net), the series of net states is thought to simulate the scalp EEG of living brains.

In this simulation several self-explanatory parameters must be set at the beginning of the program. Since the actual connectivity and strength of inhibitory or excitatory neuronal firing is determined by random numbers, the first output from the program is a comparison of the specified percentages (of callosal homotopicity, inhibition, etc.) with the actually achieved percentages. These values will differ slightly from one another depending upon the random number sequence, but will not affect the general pattern of 'EEG' activity later generated.

After reporting the statistics concerning the structure of the two cortical patches and their interconnections, the sequential firing states of the patches will be calculated. Whenever a given neuron receives excitatory input which exceeds the specified firing 'threshold', its firing potential is added to the sum total for the given patch in each cycle. The potential of that neuron is then reduced to zero for the start of summation in the next cycle. If, however, the threshold is not exceeded during the summation in each cycle, its potential is reduced only by a decay constant (specified as 0.8 in the program) and it begins summation in the following cycle with a value greater than zero. For further discussion of this method of simulation and of more realistic EEG-like results, see the literature references to Anninos and colleagues and Kohonen et al. (1977).

```
100 'SIMULATION ONE: Spatial demonstration of four callosal hypotheses
110 CONSOLE 0,25,0,1:WIDTH 80, 25:' Set up an 80-column, 25-row screen
120 DIM LH(12,12),RH(12,12),LH$(12,12),RH$(12,12)
130 PRINT"Visual pattern (0) or numbers (1)"
140 C$=INKEY$:IF C$="0" OR C$="1" THEN 150 ELSE 140
150 PRINT:PRINT" What kind of callosal effects do you want?":PRINT
160 PRINT"      1. Topographic inhibition    2. Diffuse inhibition"
170 PRINT"      3. Diffuse excitation    4. Topographic excitation"
180 A$=INKEY$:IF A$="1" OR A$="2" OR A$="3" OR A$="4" THEN 190 ELSE 180
190 CLS:PRINT"    Left Hemisphere              Right Hemisphere"
200 LOCATE 0,18:PRINT"First, two patches of cortex from the left and right
210 PRINT "         hemispheres must be constructed."
220 :
230 'Produce left and right hemisphere patches firing at background level
240 FOR A=1 TO 10:FOR B=1 TO 10:LH(A,B)=5:RH(A,B)=5:NEXT B,A
250 GOSUB *LHPRINT:GOSUB *RHPRINT
260 :
270 ' Now input left-sided engram
280 LOCATE 0,17:PRINT"Enter the coordinates of the engram:(-1,-1) to quit";
290 LOCATE 0,18:FOR A=1 TO 5:PRINT SPACE$(80);:NEXT A
300 LOCATE 10,19:PRINT USING " Activated Site No. ##)         ";N+1;
310 LOCATE 32,20:INPUT"   ";X,Y
320 IF X<0 THEN LOCATE 0,19:FOR A=1 TO 3:PRINT SPACE$(80);:NEXT A:GOTO 380
330 IF X<1 OR X>10 OR Y<1 OR Y>10 THEN GOSUB *BOUNDS:GOTO 290
340 IF LH(X,Y)>10 THEN GOSUB *USED:GOTO 290
350 IF INT(Y/2)<>Y/2 THEN LOCATE X*2,Y:PRINT"*"; ELSE LOCATE X*2+1,Y:PRINT"*";
360 LOCATE 0,19:PRINT SPACE$(80);
370 N=N+1:LH(X,Y)=LH(X,Y)+10:GOTO 290
380 GOSUB *LHSURROUND
390 GOSUB *LHPRINT
400 :
410 ' Differing right hemisphere effects depending upon callosal hypothesis:
420 IF A$="1" THEN GOSUB *MIN:       GOSUB *RHSURROUND
430 IF A$="2" THEN GOSUB *SUPPRESS:  GOSUB *RHSURROUND
440 IF A$="3" THEN GOSUB *FACILITATE: GOSUB *RHSURROUND
450 IF A$="4" THEN GOSUB *MIRROR:    GOSUB *RHSURROUND
460 GOSUB *LHPRINT:GOSUB *RHPRINT
470 FOR A=1 TO 10:FOR B=1 TO 10:RSUM=RSUM+RH(A,B):LSUM=LSUM+LH(A,B):NEXT B,A
480 LOCATE 0,16:PRINT "Total Excitation in the Two Patches is:"
490 LOCATE 0,17:FOR A=1 TO 5:PRINT SPACE$(80);:NEXT A
500 LOCATE 0,17:PRINT USING "      LH = ####    RH = ####        ";LSUM,RSUM
510 LOCATE 3,20:PRINT"Three levels of neuron activity:"
520 LOCATE 3,21:PRINT"        *    or    6,7,8 and 9 : highly active"
530 LOCATE 3,22:PRINT"        .    or          5 : background level"
540 LOCATE 3,23:PRINT"        O    or    0,1,2,3 and 4 : highly inactive";
550 IF INKEY$="" THEN 550
560 END
570 :
580 *BOUNDS
590 LOCATE 0,19:FOR A=1 TO 3:PRINT SPACE$(80);:NEXT A
600 LOCATE 0,19:PRINT"Out of bounds";:RETURN
610 :
620 *USED
630 LOCATE 0,19:FOR A=1 TO 3:PRINT SPACE$(80);:NEXT A
640 LOCATE 0,19:PRINT"Already Activated!";:RETURN
650 :
660 *MIN: ' Topographic inhibition producing mirror-mage negative pattern
670 LOCATE 0,17:FOR A= 1 TO 5:PRINT SPACE$(80);:NEXT A
680 LOCATE 0,17:PRINT" Callosal inhibition would imply decreased activity"
690 LOCATE 0,18:PRINT" at sites homotopic to active left hemisphere sites."
700 LOCATE 0,19:PRINT" Local decreases in RH surround inhibition would"
710 LOCATE 0,20:PRINT" imply relative excitation of RH surround areas."
720 LOCATE 0,22:PRINT"      The 'Mirror-Image Negative' Relationship"
730 FOR A=1 TO 10:FOR B=1 TO 10
740 IF LH(A,B)>5 THEN RH(A,B)=RH(A,B)-LH(A,B)+5
750 NEXT B,A
760 GOSUB *RHPRINT:RETURN
770 :
780 *SUPPRESS    :'Diffuse inhibition producing widespread RH deactivation
790 FOR A=1 TO 10:FOR B=1 TO 10
```

```
800 IF LH(A,B)>5 THEN RH(A,B)=RH(A,B)-4:RH(A+1,B)=RH(A+1,B)-2:RH(A+2,B)=
    RH(A+2,B)-1:RH(A-1,B)=RH(A-1,B)-2:IF A>1 THEN RH(A-2,B)=RH(A-2,B)-1
810 IF LH(A,B+1)>5 THEN RH(A,B+1)=RH(A,B+1)-2:RH(A,B+2)=RH(A,B+2)-1:RH(A,B-1)=
    RH(A,B-1)-2:IF B>1 THEN RH(A,B-2)=RH(A,B-2)-1
820 IF LH(A,B)>5 AND INT(B/2)=B/2 THEN RH(A+1,B-1)=RH(A+1,B-1)-2:RH(A+1,B+1)=
    RH(A+1,B+1)-2
830 IF LH(A,B)>5 AND INT(B/2)<>B/2 THEN RH(A-1,B-1)=RH(A-1,B-1)-2:RH(A-1,B+1)=
    RH(A-1,B+1)-2
840 NEXT B,A:GOSUB *RHPRINT:RETURN
850 :
860 *FACILITATE :'    Diffuse excitation
870 LOCATE 0,17:FOR A= 1 TO 5:PRINT SPACE$(80);:NEXT A
880 LOCATE 0,17:PRINT" Callosal excitation would imply increased activity"
890 LOCATE 0,18:PRINT" at sites homotopic to active left hemisphere sites"
900 LOCATE 0,19:PRINT"           and in surrounding RH regions."
910 FOR A=1 TO 10:FOR B=1 TO 10
920 IF LH(A,B)>5 THEN RH(A,B)=RH(A,B)+4:RH(A+1,B)=RH(A+1,B)+2:RH(A+2,B)=
    RH(A+2,B)+1:RH(A-1,B)=RH(A-1,B)+2:IF A>1 THEN RH(A-2,B)=RH(A-2,B)+1
930 IF LH(A,B)>5 THEN RH(A,B+1)=RH(A,B+1)+2:RH(A,B+2)=RH(A,B+2)+1:RH(A,B-1)=
    RH(A,B-1)+2:IF B>1 THEN RH(A,B-2)=RH(A,B-2)+1
940 IF LH(A,B)>5 AND INT(B/2)=B/2 THEN RH(A+1,B-1)=RH(A+1,B-1)+2:RH(A+1,B+1)=
    RH(A+1,B+1)+2
950 IF LH(A,B)>5 AND INT(B/2)<>B/2 THEN RH(A-1,B-1)=RH(A-1,B-1)+2:RH(A-1,B+1)=
    RH(A-1,B+1)+2
960 NEXT B,A:GOSUB *RHPRINT:RETURN
970 :
980 *MIRROR :'     Topographic (mirror-image) excitation
990 LOCATE 0,17:FOR A= 1 TO 5:PRINT SPACE$(80);:NEXT A
1000 LOCATE 0,17:PRINT "Callosal excitation would imply increased activity"
1010 LOCATE 0,19:PRINT"at sites homotopic to active in the left hemisphere."
1020 LOCATE 0,19:PRINT" Surround inhibition would produce symmetrical foci."
1030 LOCATE 0,21:PRINT "        The 'Mirror-Image' pattern"
1040 'Right hemisphere pattern
1050 FOR A=1 TO 10:FOR B=1 TO 10
1060 IF LH(A,B)>5 THEN   RH(A,B)=RH(A,B)+LH(A,B)-5
1070 NEXT B,A:GOSUB *RHPRINT:RETURN
1080 :
1090 *RHPRINT
1100 FOR X=1 TO 10:FOR Y=1 TO 9 STEP 2
1105 IF C$="1" AND RH(X,Y)>9 THEN RH(X,Y)=9
1110 IF C$="1" THEN LOCATE 53-X*2,Y:PRINT USING"#";RH(X,Y);:GOTO 1150
1120 IF RH(X,Y)<5 THEN LOCATE 53-X*2,Y:PRINT"O";
1130 IF RH(X,Y)=5 THEN LOCATE 53-X*2,Y:PRINT".";
1140 IF RH(X,Y)>5 THEN LOCATE 53-X*2,Y:PRINT"*";
1150 NEXT Y,X
1160 FOR X=1 TO 10:FOR Y=2 TO 10 STEP 2
1165 IF C$="1" AND RH(X,Y)>9 THEN RH(X,Y)=9
1170 IF C$="1" THEN LOCATE 53-X*2+1,Y:PRINT USING"#";RH(X,Y);:GOTO 1210
1180 IF RH(X,Y)<5 THEN LOCATE 52-X*2,Y:PRINT"O";
1190 IF RH(X,Y)=5 THEN LOCATE 52-X*2,Y:PRINT".";
1200 IF RH(X,Y)>5 THEN LOCATE 52-X*2,Y:PRINT"*";
1210 NEXT Y,X:RETURN
1220 :
1230 *LHPRINT
1240 FOR X=1 TO 10:FOR Y=1 TO 9 STEP 2
1245 IF C$="1" AND LH(X,Y)>9 THEN LH(X,Y)=9
1250 IF C$="1" THEN LOCATE X*2,Y:PRINT USING"#";LH(X,Y);:GOTO 1290
1260 IF LH(X,Y)<5   THEN LOCATE X*2,Y:PRINT"O";
1270 IF LH(X,Y)=5 THEN LOCATE X*2,Y:PRINT".";
1280 IF LH(X,Y)>8   THEN LOCATE X*2,Y:PRINT"*";
1290 NEXT Y,X
1300 FOR X=1 TO 10:FOR Y=2 TO 10 STEP 2
1305 IF C$="1" AND LH(X,Y)>9 THEN LH(X,Y)=9
1310 IF C$="1" THEN LOCATE X*2+1,Y:PRINT USING"#";LH(X,Y);:GOTO 1350
1320 IF LH(X,Y)<5 THEN LOCATE X*2+1,Y:PRINT"O";
1330 IF LH(X,Y)=5 THEN LOCATE X*2+1,Y:PRINT".";
1340 IF LH(X,Y)>8 THEN LOCATE X*2+1,Y:PRINT"*";
1350 NEXT Y,X:RETURN
1360 :
1370 *LHSURROUND:'    Surround inhibition in the left hemisphere
```

234

```
1380 FOR X=1 TO 10:FOR Y=1 TO 10
1390 IF LH(X+1,Y)>7    THEN LH(X,Y)=LH(X,Y)-1:'right
1400 IF LH(X-1,Y)>7    THEN LH(X,Y)=LH(X,Y)-1:'left
1410 IF LH(X,Y-1)>7    THEN LH(X,Y)=LH(X,Y)-1:'above left
1420 IF LH(X,Y+1)>7    THEN LH(X,Y)=LH(X,Y)-1:'below left
1430 IF Y/2=INT(Y/2) AND LH(X+1,Y+1)>7    THEN LH(X,Y)=LH(X,Y)-1:'below right
1440 IF Y/2=INT(Y/2) AND LH(X+1,Y-1)>7    THEN LH(X,Y)=LH(X,Y)-1:'above right
1450 IF Y/2<>INT(Y/2) AND LH(X-1,Y+1)>7    THEN LH(X,Y)=LH(X,Y)-1:'below left
1460 IF Y/2<>INT(Y/2) AND LH(X-1,Y-1)>7    THEN LH(X,Y)=LH(X,Y)-1:'above left
1470 NEXT Y,X
1480 FOR X=2 TO 9:FOR Y=2 TO 9
1490 IF LH(X+1,Y)<2    THEN LH(X,Y)=LH(X,Y)+1:'right
1500 IF LH(X-1,Y)<2    THEN LH(X,Y)=LH(X,Y)+1:'left
1510 IF LH(X,Y-1)<2    THEN LH(X,Y)=LH(X,Y)+1:'above left
1520 IF LH(X,Y+1)<2    THEN LH(X,Y)=LH(X,Y)+1:'below left
1530 IF Y/2=INT(Y/2) AND LH(X+1,Y+1)<2    THEN LH(X,Y)=LH(X,Y)+1:'below right
1540 IF Y/2=INT(Y/2) AND LH(X+1,Y-1)<2    THEN LH(X,Y)=LH(X,Y)+1:'above right
1550 IF Y/2<>INT(Y/2) AND LH(X-1,Y+1)<2    THEN LH(X,Y)=LH(X,Y)+1:'below left
1560 IF Y/2<>INT(Y/2) AND LH(X-1,Y-1)<2    THEN LH(X,Y)=LH(X,Y)+1:'above left
1570 NEXT Y,X:RETURN
1580 :
1590 *RHSURROUND: 'Surround inhibition in the right hemisphere
1600 FOR X=1 TO 10:FOR Y=1 TO 10
1610 IF RH(X+1,Y)>7    THEN RH(X,Y)=RH(X,Y)-1:'right
1620 IF RH(X-1,Y)>7    THEN RH(X,Y)=RH(X,Y)-1:'left
1630 IF RH(X,Y-1)>7    THEN RH(X,Y)=RH(X,Y)-1:'above left
1640 IF RH(X,Y+1)>7    THEN RH(X,Y)=RH(X,Y)-1:'below left
1650 IF Y/2=INT(Y/2) AND RH(X+1,Y-1)>7    THEN RH(X,Y)=RH(X,Y)-1:'above right
1660 IF Y/2=INT(Y/2) AND RH(X+1,Y+1)>7    THEN RH(X,Y)=RH(X,Y)-1:'below right
1670 IF Y/2<>INT(Y/2) AND RH(X-1,Y-1)>7    THEN RH(X,Y)=RH(X,Y)-1:'above left
1680 IF Y/2<>INT(Y/2) AND RH(X-1,Y+1)>7    THEN RH(X,Y)=RH(X,Y)-1:'below left
1690 NEXT Y,X
1700 FOR X=2 TO 9:FOR Y=2 TO 9
1710 IF RH(X+1,Y)<2    THEN RH(X,Y)=RH(X,Y)+1:'right
1720 IF RH(X-1,Y)<2    THEN RH(X,Y)=RH(X,Y)+1:'left
1730 IF RH(X,Y-1)<2    THEN RH(X,Y)=RH(X,Y)+1:'above left
1740 IF RH(X,Y+1)<2    THEN RH(X,Y)=RH(X,Y)+1:'below left
1750 IF Y/2=INT(Y/2) AND RH(X+1,Y-1)<2    THEN RH(X,Y)=RH(X,Y)+1:'above right
1760 IF Y/2=INT(Y/2) AND RH(X+1,Y+1)<2    THEN RH(X,Y)=RH(X,Y)+1:'below right
1770 IF Y/2<>INT(Y/2) AND RH(X-1,Y-1)<2    THEN RH(X,Y)=RH(X,Y)+1:'above left
1780 IF Y/2<>INT(Y/2) AND RH(X-1,Y+1)<2    THEN RH(X,Y)=RH(X,Y)+1:'below left
1790 NEXT Y,X:RETURN

100 'SIMULATION TWO: Demonstration of effects of homotopicity and inhibition
110 ' on the cyclic activity (EEG) of neural nets - ref. Anninos (1973-84)
120 DIM LH(10,200),RH(10,200): 'Maximum of 200 neurons with 10 axons each
130 DIM LFIRE(10,200),RFIRE(10,200): 'These arrays hold axonal firing.
140 DIM LSTATE(200),RSTATE(200),LEEG(200),REEG(200):' EEG arrays
150 MAX=10:MIN=-10: 'These constants denote strength of neuron firing.
160 INPUT"Generate how many 'EEG' states (<201)";CYCLES
170 INPUT"How many axons per neuron (an even number less than 11)";AXONS
180 INPUT"How many neurons in each cortical patch (<201)";NEURONS
190 INPUT"Threshold for neuron firing (2 < Threshold < 40)";THRESH
200 INPUT"Percentage of fibers which are inhibitory";INHIB:INHIB=INHIB/100
210 INPUT"Percentage of hemispheric symmetry";SYM:SYM=SYM/100
220 INPUT"Percentage of homotopic callosal fibers";HOMOT:HOMOT=HOMOT/100
230 CLS:PRINT"    Now constructing the nets."
240 :
250 ' *********    Intrahemispheric connections follow    *********
260 FOR J=1 TO NEURONS
270   CONX=CINT((AXONS/2)*RND):'No. intrahemispheric axons for each neuron
280   FOR M=1 TO CONX
290    LFIRE(M,J)=MIN+CINT((MAX-MIN)*RND):'Strength of neuron firing
300    IF INHIB>RND THEN LFIRE(M,J)=-1*ABS(LFIRE(M,J)) ELSE LFIRE(M,J)=
       ABS(LFIRE(M,J)):' Determine excitatory or inhibitory nature
310    IF SYM>RND THEN RFIRE(M,J)=LFIRE(M,J):T=1 ELSE IF INHIB>RND THEN
       RFIRE(M,J)=-1*ABS(MIN+CINT((MAX-MIN)*RND)):T=0 ELSE RFIRE(M,J)=
       ABS(MIN+CINT((MAX-MIN)*RND)):T=0:'Determine symmetry
320    LH(M,J)=CINT(NEURONS*RND):'Determine destination of LH axons
330    IF T=1 THEN RH(M,J)=LH(M,J) ELSE RH(M,J)=CINT(NEURONS*RND)
340   NEXT M,J
```

235

```
350 :
360 ' ************    Callosal connections follow    *************
370 FOR J=1 TO NEURONS
380  CONX=AXONS/2+CINT(AXONS/2*RND):'Determine no. of callosal axons
390  FOR M=AXONS/2+1 TO CONX
400   LFIRE(M,J)=MIN+CINT((MAX-MIN)*RND):FLAG=1
410   IF INHIB>RND(I) THEN LFIRE(M,J)=-1*ABS(LFIRE(M,J)) ELSE LFIRE(M,J)=
      ABS(LFIRE(M,J)):'Set firing strength
420   LH(M,J)=CINT(NEURONS*RND):'Determine axonal destinations
430   IF HOMOT>RND THEN RH(M,J)=LH(M,J):RFIRE(M,J)=LFIRE(M,J) ELSE RH(M,J)
      =CINT(NEURONS*RND):RFIRE(M,J)=MIN+CINT((MAX-MIN)*RND):FLAG=0
440   IF FLAG=0 THEN RFIRE(M,J)=-1*ABS(RFIRE(M,J)):IF INHIB<RND THEN
      RFIRE(M,J)=ABS(RFIRE(M,J))
450 NEXT M,J
460 :
470 ' **********    Count excitation and inhibition    **********
480 FOR J=1 TO NEURONS:FOR M=1 TO AXONS/2
490   IF LFIRE(M,J)>0 THEN LASSEX=LASSEX+1:' Left Association Excitatory
500   IF LFIRE(M,J)<0 THEN LASSIN=LASSIN+1:' Left Association Inhibitory
510   IF LFIRE(M,J)>0 THEN RASSEX=RASSEX+1:' Right Association Excitatory
520   IF LFIRE(M,J)<0 THEN RASSIN=RASSIN+1:' Right Association Inhibitory
530 IF LH(M,J)=RH(M,J) AND LH(M,J)<>0 THEN SF=SF+2:' Symmetrical fibers
540 NEXT M,J
550 FOR J=1 TO NEURONS:FOR M=AXONS/2+1 TO AXONS
560   IF LFIRE(M,J)>0 THEN EXCAL12=EXCAL12+1:' Excitatory Callosal (L->R)
570   IF LFIRE(M,J)<0 THEN INCAL12=INCAL12+1:' Inhibitory Callosal (L->R)
580   IF RFIRE(M,J)>0 THEN EXCAL21=EXCAL21+1:' Excitatory Callosal (R->L)
590   IF RFIRE(M,J)<0 THEN INCAL21=INCAL21+1:' Inhibitory Callosal (R->L)
600   IF LH(M,J)=RH(M,J) AND LH(M,J)<>0 THEN HF=HF+2:'Homotopic fibers
610 NEXT M,J
620 TOTEX=LASSEX+EXCAL21+RASSEX+EXCAL12:' Total No. of Excitatory Fibers
630 TOTIN=LASSIN+INCAL21+RASSIN+INCAL12:' Total No. of Inhibitory Fibers
640 TOTCAL=EXCAL12+EXCAL21+INCAL12+INCAL21:' Total No. of Callosal Fibers
650 PCNTHOM=100*HF/TOTCAL:INHIBPCNT=100*TOTIN/(TOTIN+TOTEX)
660 TOTFIB=LASSEX+LASSIN+RASSEX+RASSIN:PCNTSYM=100*SF/TOTFIB
670 LEX=LASSEX+EXCAL21:REX=RASSEX+EXCAL12
680 LIN=LASSIN+INCAL21:RIN=RASSIN+INCAL12
690 :
700 CLS: ' ******************    Print Results    ******************
710 PRINT USING"Homotopicity Wanted ### & Achieved ###";HOMOT*100,PCNTHOM
720 PRINT USING"    Symmetry Wanted ### & Achieved ###";SYM*100,PCNTSYM
730 PRINT USING"    Inhibition Wanted ### & Achieved ###";INHIB*100,INHIBPCNT
740 PRINT:PRINT"  NATURE OF CONNECTIONS    EXCITATORY  INHIBITORY"
750 PRINT"------------------------------------------------------------"
760 PRINT USING" Left associative fibers    ####        ####";LASSEX,LASSIN
770 PRINT USING"Right associative fibers    ####        ####";RASSEX,RASSIN
780 PRINT USING"    R->L callosal fibers    ####        ####";EXCAL21,INCAL21
790 PRINT USING"    L->R callosal fibers    ####        ####";EXCAL12,INCAL12
800 PRINT USING"       Total left fibers    ####        ####";LEX,LIN
810 PRINT USING"      Total right fibers    ####        ####";REX,RIN
820 :
830 ' *****  Add the Effects of Consecutive Cycles to Find the 'EEG'  *****
840 PRINT:PRINT"    Now calculating 'EEG' changes over";CYCLES;"cycles."
850 DECAY=.8: ' The decay is the percentage carry-from from state to state.
860 FOR K=1 TO CYCLES:FOR J=1 TO NEURONS:FOR M=1 TO AXONS
870    LSTATE(LH(M,J))=LSTATE(LH(M,J))+LFIRE(M,J)
880    RSTATE(RH(M,J))=RSTATE(RH(M,J))+RFIRE(M,J)
890    NEXT M:FOR M=AXONS/2+1 TO AXONS
900    LSTATE(RH(M,J))=LSTATE(RH(M,J))+RFIRE(M,J)
910    RSTATE(LH(M,J))=RSTATE(LH(M,J))+LFIRE(M,J)
920   NEXT M,J
930   ************    Summation for EEG    *************
940   FOR J=1 TO NEURONS
950    IF LSTATE(J)>THRESH THEN LEEG=LEEG+LSTATE(J):LSTATE(J)=0 ELSE
       LSTATE(J)=CINT(DECAY*LSTATE(J))
960    IF RSTATE(J)>THRESH THEN REEG=REEG+RSTATE(J):RSTATE(J)=0 ELSE
       LSTATE(J)=CINT(DECAY*LSTATE(J))
970    NEXT J
980   LEEG(K)=LEEG:REEG(K)=REEG:LEEG=0:REEG=0
990   PRINT K,LEEG(K),REEG(K)
1000 NEXT K
```

References

Abeles, M. (1982) *Local Cerebral Circuits: An Electrophysiological Study*, Berlin, Springer.

Abercrombie, M. L. J., Lindon, R. L. and Tyson, M. C. (1964) 'Associated movement in normal and physically handicapped children,' *Developmental Medicine and Child Neurology*, 6, 573–80.

Achim, A. and Corballis, M. C. (1977) 'Mirror-image equivalence and the anterior commissure,' *Neuropsychologia*, 15, 475–8.

Angevine, J. B., Locke, S. and Yakovlev, P. I. (1962) 'Limbic nuclei of thalamus and connections of limbic cortex (IV),' *Archives of Neurology*, 7, 518–28.

Anninos, P. A. (1972) 'Cyclic modes in artificial neural nets', *Kybernetik*, 11, 5–14.

Anninos, P. A. and Cook, N. D. (1986) 'Computer simulation of the corpus callosum,' *Biological Cybernetics*, (in press).

Anninos, P. A. and Cyrulink, R. A. (1977) 'A neural net model for epilepsy', *Journal of Theoretical Biology*, 66, 695–709.

Anthony, R. J. (1938) 'Essai de recherche d'une expression anatomique approximative du degré d'organisation cerebrale autre que le poids de l'encephale comparée au poids du corps,' *Bulletin de la Societé d'Anthropologie de Paris*, 9, 1–67.

Bailey, P. and von Bonin, G. (1951) *The Isocortex of Man*, Urbana, University of Illinois Press.

Bava, A., Fadiga, E., Manzoni, T. and Maricchi, M. (1970) 'Inhibitory interactions between thalamic VLP nuclei of two sides,' *Archives Italienne Biologie*, 108, 462–73.

Beaumont, J. G. (1982) 'Studies with verbal stimuli,' in Beaumont, J. G. (ed.) *Divided Visual Field Studies of Cerebral Organization*, New York, Academic Press, 67–86.

Berlucchi, G. (1981) 'Interhemispheric asymmetries in visual discriminations: a neurophysiological hypothesis,' *Documenta Ophthalmologica Proceedings Series*, 30, 87–93.

Berlucchi, G. (1983) 'Two hemispheres but one brain,' *Behavioral and Brain Sciences*, 6, 171–3.

Blinkov, S. M. and Glezer, I. I. (1968) *The Human Brain in Figures and Tables*, New York, Plenum Press.

Bogen, J. E. (1979) 'The callosal syndrome,' in Heilman, K. M. and

Valenstein, E. (eds) *Clinical Neuropsychology*, New York, Oxford University Press, 308–59.

Bradshaw, J. L. and Nettleton, N. C. (1983) *Human Cerebral Asymmetry*, Englewood Cliffs, NJ, Prentice-Hall.

Braitenberg, V. (1977) 'The concept of symmetry in neuroanatomy,' *Annals of the New York Academy of Sciences*, 299, 186–96.

Brownell, H. H., Michel, D., Powelson, J. and Gardner, H. (1983) 'Surprise but not coherence: sensitivity to verbal humor in right-hemisphere patients,' *Brain and Language*, 18, 20–7.

Brownell, H. H., Potter, H. H., Michelow, D. and Gardner, H. (1984) 'Sensitivity to lexical denotation and connotation in brain-damaged patients: a double dissociation?,' *Brain and Language*, 22, 253–65.

Bruner, J. S. (1968) *Processes of Cognitive Growth: Infancy*, vol. 3, Worcester, Mass., Clark University Press.

Bunge, M. (1959) *Metascientific Queries*, Springfield, Ill., C. C. Thomas.

Burkland, C. W. and Smith, A. (1977) 'Language and the cerebral hemispheres,' *Neurology*, 27, 627–33.

Butler, S. R. (1968) 'A memory-record for visual discrimination habits produced in both cerebral hemispheres of monkey when only one has received direct visual information,' *Brain Research*, 10, 152–67.

Butler, S. R. (1979) 'Interhemispheric transfer of visual information via corpus callosum and anterior commissure in the monkey,' in Russell, I. S. *et al.* (eds) *Structure and Function of the Cerebral Commissures*, New York, Macmillan, 343–57.

Campbell, A. L., Bogen, J. E. and Smith, A. (1981) 'Disorganization and reorganization of cognitive and sensorimotor functions in cerebral commissurotomy,' *Brain*, 104, 493–511.

Caramazza, A., Gordon, J., Zurif, E. G. and DeLuca, D. (1976) 'Right hemisphere damage and verbal problem solving behavior,' *Brain and Language*, 3, 41–6.

Cavalli, M., DeRenzi, E., Faglioni, P. and Vitale, A. (1981) 'Impairment of right brain-damaged patients on a linguistic cognitive task,' *Cortex*, 17, 545–56.

Chiarello, C. (1980) 'A house divided? Cognitive functioning with callosal agenesis,' *Brain and Language*, 11, 128–58.

Claridge, G. S. and Broks, P. (1984) 'Schizotypy and hemisphere function,' *Personality Theory and Individual Differences*, 4, 119–35.

Collins, R. L. (1977) 'Toward an admissable genetic model for the inheritance of the degree and direction of asymmetry,' in Harnad, S. *et al.* (eds) *Lateralization in the Nervous System*, New York, Academic Press, 137–50.

Coltheart, M. (1983) 'The right hemisphere and disorders of reading' in Young, A. W. (ed.) *Functions of the Right Cerebral Hemisphere*, New York, Academic Press, 173–202.

Cook, N. D. (1977) 'The case for reverse translation,' *Journal of Theoretical Biology*, 64, 113–32.

Cook, N. D. (1979) 'Systemic stability and flexibility,' *Journal of Social and Biological Structures*, 2, 315–32.

Cook, N. D. (1980a) 'An isomorphism of control in natural, social and cybernetic systems,' *Journal of Cybernetics*, 10, 29–39.

Cook, N. D. (1980b) *Stability and Flexibility: An Analysis of Natural Systems*, Oxford, Pergamon Press.

Cook, N. D. (1984a) 'Homotopic callosal inhibition,' *Brain and Language*, 14, 123–44.

Cook, N. D. (1984b) 'Callosal inhibition: the key to the brain code,' *Behavioral Science*, 26, 234–55.

Cook, N. D. (1984c) 'The transmission of information in natural systems,' *Journal of Theoretical Biology*, 133, 142–65.

Corballis, M. C. and Beale, I. L. (1976) *The Psychology of Left and Right*, Hillsdale, NJ, Erlbaum.

Corballis, M. C. and Morgan, M. J. (1978) 'On the biological basis of human laterality,' *Behavioral and Brain Sciences*, 1, 261–9.

Creutzfeldt, O. D. (1975) 'Some problems of cortical organization in the light of ideas of the classical 'Hirnpathologie' and of modern neurophysiology' in Zulch, K. J. and Creutzfeldt, O. D. (eds) *Cerebral Localization*, Berlin, Springer Verlag, 217–26.

Creutzfeldt, O. D. (1977) 'Generality of the functional structure of the neocortex,' *Naturwissenschaften*, 64, 507–17.

Crick, F. (1979) 'Thinking about the brain,' *Scientific American*, Nov., 181–8.

Crick, F. (1984) 'Functions of the thalamic reticular complex – the searchlight hypothesis,' *Proceedings of the National Academy of Sciences* (USA), 81, 4586–90.

Critchley, M. (1928) *Mirror-writing*, London, Kegan Paul.

Davidoff, J. (1982) 'Studies with non-verbal stimuli,' in Beaumont, J. G. (ed.) *Divided Visual Field Studies of Cerebral Organization*, New York, Academic Press.

Delis, D. C., Wapner, W., Gardner, H. and Moses, J. A. (1983) 'The contribution of the right hemisphere to the organization of paragraphs,' *Cortex*, 19, 43–50.

Denenberg, V. H. (1980) 'General systems theory, brain organization and early experience,' *American Journal of Physiology: Regulatory, Integrative and Comparative Physiology*, 238, 213–23.

Denenberg, V. H. (1981) 'Hemispheric laterality in animals and the effects of early experience,' *Behavioral and Brain Sciences*, 4, 1–49.

Denenberg, V. H. (1983) 'Micro and macro theories of the brain,' *Behavioral and Brain Sciences*, 6, 174–8.

Denning, H. (1966) *Lehrbuch der Inneren Medizin*, Band II, 7 Aufl., Stuttgart, Georg Thieme.

Dennis, M. (1976) 'Impaired sensory and motor differentiation with corpus callosum agenesis: a lack of callosal inhibition during ontogeny?,' *Neuropsychologia*, 14, 455–69.

Dimond, S. J. (1972) *The Double Brain*, London, Churchill Livingstone.

Dimond, S. J. (1977) 'Evolution and lateralization of the brain: concluding remarks,' *Annals of the New York Academy of Sciences*, 299, 477–501.

Dimond, S. J. (1979a) 'Symmetry and asymmetry in the vertebrate brain,' in Oakley, D. A. and Plotkin, H. C. (eds) *Brain, Behaviour and Evolution*, London, Methuen, 189–218.

Dimond, S. J. (1979b) 'Disconnection and psychopathology,' in Gruzelier, J. and Flor-Henry, P. (eds) *Hemisphere Asymmetries of Function in Psychopathology*, Amsterdam, Elsevier, 35–46.

Donchin, E., Kutas, M. and McCarthy, G. (1977) 'Electrocortical indices of hemispheric utilization,' in Harnad, S. *et al.* (eds) *Lateralization in the Nervous System*, New York, Academic Press, 339–84.

Doty, R. W. and Negrao, N. (1973) 'Forebrain commissures and vision,' in Jung, R. (ed.) *Handbook of Sensory Physiology*, vol. VII/3B, Berlin, Springer, 543–82.

Doty, R. W. and Overman, W. H. (1977) 'Mnemonic role of forebrain commissures in macaques,' in Harnad, S. *et al.* (eds) *Lateralization in the Nervous System*, New York, Academic Press, 75–88.

Doty, R. W., Overman, W. H. and Negrao, N. (1979) 'Role of forebrain commissures in hemispheric specialization and memory in macaques,' in Russell, I. S. *et al.* (eds) *Structure and Function of the Cerebral Commissures*, New York, Macmillan, 333–42.

Doty, R. W., Yamaga, K. and Negrao, N. (1973) 'The unilateral engram,' *Acta Neurobiologica Experimentalis*, 33, 711–28.

Dumas, R. and Morgan, A. (1975) 'EEG asymmetry as a function of occupation, task and task difficult,' *Neuropsychologia*, 13, 219–28.

Eccles, J. C. (1977) *The Self and its Brain*, Berlin, Springer.

Elias, H. and Schwartz, D. (1969) 'Surface areas of the cerebral cortex of mammals determined by stereological methods,' *Science*, 166, 111–13.

Elliot, F. A. (1969) 'The corpus callosum, cingulate gyrus, septum pellucidum, septal area and fornix,' *Handbook of Clinical Neurology*, 2, 758–75.

Enge, H. A. (1966) *Introduction to Nuclear Physics*, Reading, Mass., Addison-Wesley, 81.

Ettlinger, E. G. (ed.) (1965) *Functions of the Corpus Callosum*, London, Churchill Livingstone.

Ferriss, G. S. and Dorsen, M. M. (1975) 'Agenesis of the corpus callosum: I. Neuropsychological studies,' *Cortex*, 11, 95–122.

Fleischhauer, K. and Wartenberg, H. (1967) 'Elektronmikroskopische Untersuchungen über das Wachstum der Nerverfassern und über das Auftreten von Markschelden im Corpus Callosum der Katze'. *Zeitschrift für Zellforschung*, 83, 568–81.

Flor-Henry, P. (1979a) 'On certain aspects of the localization of the cerebral systems regulating and determining emotion,' *Biological Psychiatry*, 14, 677–98.

Flor-Henry, P. (1979b) 'Laterality, shifts of cerebral dominance, sinistrality and psychosis,' in Gruzelier, G. H. and Flor-Henry, P. (eds) *Hemispheric Asymmetries of Function in Psychopathology*, Amsterdam, Elsevier/North Holland, 3–19.

Flor-Henry, P. (1983) *Cerebral Basis of Psychopathology*, Boston, Mass., Wright.

French, J. D. (1973) 'The reticular formation,' in Fields, J., Magoun, H. and Hall, W. (eds) *Handbook of Physiology*, sect. 1, vol. 2, Washington, DC, American Physiological Society, 1281–1305.

Gainotti, G., Caltagirone, C. and Miceli, G. (1983) 'Selective impairment of semantic–lexical discrimination in right-brain-damaged patients,' in Perecman, E. (ed.) *Cognitive Processing of the Right Hemisphere*, New York, Academic Press, 149–68.

Galaburda, A. M. (1984) 'Anatomical asymmetries,' in Galaburda, A. M. and Geschwind, N. (eds) *Cerebral Dominance: The Biological Foundations*, Cambridge, Mass., Harvard University Press, 11–25.

Galaburda, A. M., LeMay, M., Kemper, T. L. and Geschwind, N. (1978) 'Right–left asymmetries of the brain,' *Science*, 199, 852–6.

Galin, D. (1977) 'Lateral specializations and psychiatric issues: speculations on development and the evolution of consciousness,' *Annals of the New York Academy of Sciences*, 299, 397–411.

Galin, D. and Ellis, R. R. (1975) 'Asymmetry in evoked potentials as an index of lateralized cognitive processes: relation to EEG alpha asymmetry,' *Neuropsychologia*, 3, 45–50.

Gardner, H., Brownell, H., Wapner, W. and Michelow, D. (1983) 'Missing the point: the role of the right hemisphere in the processing of complex linguistic materials,' in Perecman, E. (ed.) *Cognitive Processing in the Right Hemisphere*, New York, Academic Press, 169–92.

Gardner, H. and Denes, G. (1973) 'Connotative judgments by aphasic patients on a pictorial adaptation of the semantic differential,' *Cortex*, 9, 183–96.

Gardner, H., Ling, K., Flamm, L. and Silverman, J. (1975) 'Comprehension and appreciation of humor in brain-damaged patients,' *Brain*, 98, 399–412.

Garey, L. J. (1979) 'Mammalian neocortical commissures,' in Russell, I. S. *et al.* (eds) *Structure and Function of the Cerebral Commissures*, New York, Macmillan, 147–54.

Gazzaniga, M. S. (1970) *The Bisected Brain*, New York, Appleton-Century-Crofts.

Gazzaniga, M. S. and LeDoux, J. (1978) *The Integrated Mind*, New York, Plenum Press.

Gazzaniga, M. S., Volpe, B. T., Smylie, C. S., Wilson, D. H. and LeDoux, J. E. (1979) 'Plasticity in speech organization following commissurotomy,' *Brain*, 102, 805–15.

Geschwind, N. (1965) 'Disconnexion syndrome in animals and man,' *Brain*, 88, 237–94, 585–644.

Geschwind, N. (1982) 'Disorders of attention: a frontier in neuropsychology,' *Philosophical Transactions of the Royal Society* (London), B298, 173–85.

Geschwind, N. and Galaburda, A. M. (eds) (1984) *Cerebral Dominance: The Biological Foundations*, Cambridge, Mass., Harvard University Press.

Geschwind, N. and Kaplan, E. (1962) 'The corpus callosum syndrome,' *Neurology*, 12, 675–85.

Geschwind, N. and Levitsky, W. (1968) 'Human brain: left–right asymmetries in temporal speech region,' *Science*, 161, 186–7.

Gevins, A. S., Zeitlin, G. M., Doyle, J. C., Schaffer, R. E. and Callaway, E. (1979) 'EEG patterns during 'cognitive' tasks. II. Analysis of controlled tasks,' *Electroencephalography and Clinical Neurophysiology*, 47, 704–10.

Goldman, P. S. and Nauta, W. J. H. (1977) 'Columnar distribution of cortico-cortical fibers in prefrontal association, limbic and motor cortex of the developing rhesus monkey,' *Brain Research*, 122, 393–415.

Goldman-Rakic, P. S. (1984) 'Modular organization of prefrontal cortex,' *Trends in the Neurosciences*, Nov., 419–24.

Goldman-Rakic, P. S. and Schwartz, M. L. (1982) 'Interdigitation of contralateral and ipsilateral columnar projections to frontal cortex in primates,' *Science*, 216, 755–7.

Gordon, H. W. (1974) Auditory specialization of the right and left hemispheres, in Kinsbourne, M. and Smith, W. L. (eds) *Hemispheric Disconnection and Cerebral Function*, Springfield, Ill., C. C. Thomas, 126–36.

Gott, P. S. (1973) 'Cognitive abilities following right and left hemispherectomy,' *Cortex*, 9, 266–74.

Gruzelier, G. H. and Flor-Henry, P. (eds) (1979) *Hemispheric Asymmetries of Function in Psychopathology*, Amsterdam, Elsevier/North Holland.

Guiard, Y. (1980) 'Cerebral hemispheres and selective attention,' *Acta Psychologica*, 46, 41–61.

Gur, R. C., Gur, R. E., Rosen, A. D., Warach, S., Alavi, A., Greenberg, J. and Reivich, M. (1983) 'A cognitive-motor network demonstrated by positron emission tomography,' *Neuropsychologia*, 21, 601–6.

Gur, R. C., Packer, I. K., Hungerbuhler, J. D., Reivich, M., Obrist, W. D., Amarnek, W. S. and Sackheim, H. A. (1980) 'Differences in distribution of grey and white matter in human cerebral hemisphere,' *Science*, 207, 1226–8.

Hamilton, C. R. (1977) 'Investigation of perceptual and mnemonic lateralization in monkeys,' in Harnad, S. *et al.* (eds) *Lateralization in the Nervous System*, New York, Academic Press, 45–62.

Harrington, A. (1986) 'Nineteenth-century ideas on hemisphere differences and "duality of mind",' *Behavioral and Brain Sciences* 8, 617–60.

Hatta, T. (1981) 'Differential processing of Kanji and Kana stimuli in Japanese people: some implications from Stroop-test results,' *Neuropsychologia*, 19, 87–93.

Hedreen, J. C. and Yin, T. C. T. (1981) 'Homotopic and heterotopic callosal afferents of caudal inferior parietal lobule in *Macaca mulatta*,' *Journal of Comparative Neurology*, 197, 605–21.

Heilman, K. M., Scholes, R. and Watson, R. T. (1975) 'Auditory affective agnosia,' *Journal of Neurology, Neurosurgery and Psychiatry*, 38, 9–72.

Henneberg, R. (1910) 'Messung der Oberflachenausdehnung der Grosshirnrinde,' *Journal für Psychologie und Neurologie*, 17, 144–58.

Hess, P., Negishi, K. and Creutzfeldt, O. (1975) 'The horizontal spread of intracortical inhibition in the visual cortex,' *Experimental Brain Research*, 27, 415–19.

Hofman, M. A. (1983) 'Encephalization in hominids,' *Brain, Behavior and Evolution*, 22, 102–13.

Hossman, K. A. (1975) 'Transcallosal potentials in the corpus callosum of the cat,' in Zulch, K. J., Creutzfeldt, O. D. and Galbraith, G. C. (eds) *Cerebral Localization*, Berlin, Springer, 150–7.

Hrbek, J. (1976) 'The basic physiological mechanisms of nervous integration,' *Acta Universitatis Palackianae Olomucensis*, 77, 5–23.

Hubel, D. H. and Wiesel, T. N. (1977) 'Functional architecture of monkey visual cortex,' *Proceedings of the Royal Society of London*, B198, 1–59.

Hunt, M. (1982) *The Universe Within*, London, Harvester Press.

Iwata, M., Sugishita, M. and Toyokura, Y. (1982) in Katsuki, S., *et al.* (eds) *Neurology*, Amsterdam, Excerpta Medica, 53–62.

Jacobson, S. and Marcus, E. M. (1970) 'The laminar distribution of the corpus callosum: a comparative study in the rat, cat, rhesus monkey and chimpanzee,' *Brain Research*, 24, 513–20.

Jaynes, J. (1976) *The Origin of Consciousness in the Breakdown of the Bicameral Mind*, Boston, Mass., Houghton & Mifflin.

Jerison, H. J. (1973) *Evolution of the Brain and Intelligence*, New York, Academic Press.

Jones, E. G., Burton, H. and Porter, R. (1975) 'Commissural and cortico-cortical "columns" in the somatic sensory cortex of primates,' *Science*, 190, 572–4.

Jones, E. G. and Powell, T. P. S. (1970) 'An anatomical study of converging sensory pathways within the cerebral cortex of the monkey,' *Brain*, 93, 793–820.

Jones, R. K. (1966) 'Observations on stammering after localized cerebral injury,' *Journal of Neurology, Neurosurgery and Psychiatry*, 29, 192–5.

Kinsbourne, M. (1974) 'Lateral interaction in the brain,' in Kinsbourne, M. and Smith, W. L. (eds) *Hemispheric Disconnection and Cerebral Function*, Springfield, Ill., C. C. Thomas, 239–59.

Kinsbourne, M. (1978) *Asymmetrical Function of the Brain*, New York, Academic Press.

Kinsbourne, M. (1982) 'Hemispheric specialization and the growth of human understanding,' *American Psychologist*, 37, 411–20.

Knopman, D. S., Rubens, A. B., Klassen, A. C. and Meyer, M. W. (1982) 'Regional cerebral blood flow correlates of auditory processing,' *Archives of Neurology*, 39, 487–93.

Kohonen, T., Lehtio, P., Rovamo, J., Hyvarinen, J., Bry, K. and Vainio, L. A. (1977) 'Principle of neural associative memory,' *Neuroscience*, 2, 1065–76.

Kuhn, T. S. (1970) *The Structure of Scientific Revolutions*, 2nd edn, Chicago, Chicago University Press.

LaCroix, J. M. and Comper, P. (1979) 'Asymmetric galvanic skin responses to verbal and non-verbal stimuli in man,' *Psychophysiology*, 16, 116–24.

Larsen, B., Skinhoj, E. and Lassen, N. A. (1978) 'Variations in regional cortical blood flow in the right and left hemispheres during automatic speech,' *Brain*, 101, 193–209.

Lassen, N. A., Ingvar, D. H., and Skinhoj, E., 'Brain function and blood flow', *Scientific American*, No. 4, 50.

Laszlo, E. (1973) *Introduction to General Systems Philosophy*, New York, Braziller.

LeMay, M. (1976) 'Morphological cerebral asymmetries of modern man, fossil man and non-human primates,' *Annals of the New York Academy of Sciences*, 280, 349–66.

LeMay, M. and Culebras, A. (1972) 'Human brain – morphologic differences in the hemispheres demonstrated by carotid arteriography,' *New England Journal of Medicine*, 287, 168–70.

Lesser, R. (1974) 'Verbal comprehension in aphasia: an English version of three Italian tests,' *Cortex*, 10, 247–63.

Ley, R. G. and Bryden, M. P. (1979) 'Hemispheric differences in processing emotions and faces,' *Brain and Language*, 7, 127–36.

Liberman, A. M., Cooper, F., Shankweiler, D. and Studdert-Kennedy, M. (1967) 'Perception of the speech code,' *Psychological Review*, 74, 431–61.

Lorente de No, R. (1938) 'Cerebral cortex: architecture, intracortical connections and motor projections,' in Fulton, J. F. (ed.) *Physiology of the Nervous System*, Oxford, Oxford University Press, 291–339.

Mandell, A. J. and Knapp, S. (1979) 'Asymmetry and mood, emergent properties of serotonin regulation,' *Archives of General Psychiatry*, 36, 909–16.

Marshall, J. C. (1981) 'Hemispheric specialization: what, how and when,' *Behavioral and Brain Sciences*, 4, 72–3.

Maximilian, V. A. (1982) 'Cortical blood flow asymmetries during monaural verbal stimulation,' *Brain and Language*, 15, 1–11.

Mazziotta, J. C., Phelps, M. E., Carson, R. E. and Kuhl, D. E. (1982) 'Tomographic mapping of human cerebral metabolism: auditory stimulation,' *Neurology* (Minneapolis), 32, 921–37.

Mekler, L. B. (1967) 'Mechanism of biological memory,' *Nature*, 215, 481–4.

Mellish, C. S. (1985) *Computer Interpretation of Natural Language Descriptions*, New York, John Wiley.

Merzenich, M. M. and Kaas, J. H. (1980) 'Principles of organization of sensory-perceptual systems in mammals,' *Progress in Psychobiology and Physiological Psychology*, 9, 1–42.

Mesulam, M. M. (1981) 'A cortical network for directed attention and unilateral neglect,' *Annals of Neurology*, 10, 309–25.

Middlebrooks, J. C., Dykes, R. W. and Merzenich, M. M. (1980) 'Binaural response-specific bands in primary auditory cortex of the cat: topographical organization orthogonal to isofrequency contours,' *Brain Research*, 181, 31–48.

Milner, A. D. (1983) 'Neuropsychological studies of callosal agenesis,' *Psychological Medicine*, 13, 721–5.

Milner, A. D. and Jeeves, M. A. (1979) 'A review of behavioral studies of agenesis of the corpus callosum,' in Russell, I. S. *et al.* (eds) *Structure and Function of the Cerebral Commissures*, New York, Macmillan, 428–48.

Mitchell, D. E. and Blakemore, C. (1970) 'Binocular depth perception and the corpus callosum,' *Vision Research*, 10, 49–54.

Moscovitch, M. (1973) 'Language and the cerebral hemispheres: reaction time studies and their implications for models of cerebral dominance,' in Pliner, P., Alloway, T. and Krames, L. (eds) *Communication and Affect: Language and Thought*, New York, Academic Press, 89–126.

Mountcastle, V. B. (1978) 'An organizing principle for cerebral function: the unit module and the distributed system,' in Edelman, G. M. and Mountcastle, V. B. (eds) *The Mindful Brain*, Cambridge, Mass., MIT Press, 7–50.

Myers, R. E. (1965) 'The neocortical commissures and interhemispheric transmission of information,' in Ettlinger, E. G. (ed.) *Functions of the Corpus Callosum*, London, Churchill Livingstone, 1–17.

Nauta, W. J. H. and Haymaker, W. (1969) 'Hypothalamic nuclei and fiber connections,' in Haymaker, W., *et al.* (eds) *The Hypothalamus*, Springfield, Ill., C. C. Thomas, 136–209.

Nebes, R. D. (1974) 'Hemispheric specialization in commissurotomized man,' *Psychological Bulletin*, 81, 1–14.

Nieuwenhuys, R., Voogd, S. and vanHuijzen, C. (1978) *The Human Central Nervous System*, Berlin, Springer.

Noble, J. (1966) 'Mirror-images and the forebrain commissures of the monkey,' *Nature*, 211, 1263–5.

Noble, J. (1968) 'Paradoxical interocular transfer of mirror-image discrimination in the optic chiasm-sectioned monkey,' *Brain Research*, 10, 127–51.

Nottebohm, F. (1977) 'Asymmetries of neural control of vocalization in the canary,' in Harnad, S. *et al.* (eds) *Lateralization in the Nervous System*, New York, Academic Press, 23–44.

Ojemann, G. A. (1983) 'The intrahemispheric organization of human language, derived with electrical stimulation techniques,' *Trends in the Neurosciences*, May, 184–9.

Oke, A., Keller, R., Mefford, I. and Adams, R. N. (1978) 'Lateralization of norepinephrine in human thalamus,' *Science*, 200, 1411–3.

Ornstein, R. E. (1972) *The Psychology of Consciousness*, San Francisco, Calif., Freeman.

Orton, S. T. (1937) *Reading, Writing and Speech Problems in Children*, London, Chapman & Hall.

Passingham, R. E. (1981) 'Broca's area and the origin of human vocal skills,' *Philosophical Transactions of the Royal Society of London*, B292, 167–75.

Payne, B. R., Pearson, H. E. and Berman, N. (1984) 'Role of the corpus callosum in functional organization of cat striate cortex,' *Journal of Neurophysiology*, 52, 570–94.

Penfield, W. (1959) *Speech and Brain Mechanisms*, Princeton, NJ, Princeton University Press.

Phillips, C. G., Zeki, S. and Barlow, H. B. (1984) 'Localization of function in the cerebral cortex,' *Brain*, 107, 328–60.

Prohovnik, I., Hakansson, K. and Risberg, J. (1980) 'Observations on the functional significance of regional blood flow in "resting" normal subjects,' *Neuropsychologia*, 18, 203–17.

Rakic, P. and Yakovlev, P. I. (1968) 'Development of the corpus callosum and the cavum septi in man,' *Journal of Comparative Neurology*, 132, 45–72.

Reeves, A. G. (ed.) (1985) *Epilepsy and the Corpus Callosum*, New York, Plenum Press.

Regard, M. and Landis, T. (1984) 'Experimentally induced semantic paralexias in normals: a property of the right hemisphere,' *Cortex*, 20, 263–70.

Robinson, D. L. (1983) 'An analysis of human EEG responses in the alpha range of frequencies,' *International Journal of Neuroscience*, 22, 81–98.

Rockel, A. J., Hiorns, R. W. and Powell, T. P. S. (1980) 'The basic uniformity in the fine structure of the neocortex,' *Brain*, 103, 221–44.

Ross, E. D. and Mesulam, M. M. (1979) 'Dominant language functions of the right hemisphere,' *Archives of Neurology*, 36, 144–8.

Rubens, A. B. (1977) 'Anatomical asymmetries of human cerebral cortex,' in Harnad, S. *et al.* (eds) *Lateralization in the Nervous System*, New York, Academic Press, 503–16.

Russell, I. S., Van Hof, M. W. and Berlucchi, G. (eds) (1979) *Structure and Function of the Cerebral Commissures*, New York, Macmillan, 181–94.

Sasanuma, S., Itoh, M., Kobayashi, Y. and Mori, K. (1980) 'The nature of the task–stimulus interaction in the tachistoscopic recognition of Kana and Kanji words,' *Brain and Language*, 9, 298–306.

Saul, R. E. and Sperry, R. W. (1968) 'Absence of commissurotomy symptoms with agenesis of the corpus callosum,' *Neurology*, 18, 307–13.

Schott, G. D. (1980) 'Mirror movements of the left arm following peripheral damage to the preferred right arm,' *Journal of Neurology, Neurosurgery and Psychiatry*, 43, 768–73.

Segre, E. (1977) *Nuclei and Particles*, 2nd edn, Reading, Mass., W. A. Benjamin, 748–800.

Selnes, O. A. (1974) 'The corpus callosum: some anatomical and functional considerations with special reference to language,' *Brain and Language*, 1, 111–39.

Shephard, G. M. (1974) *The Synaptic Organization of the Brain*, Oxford, Oxford University Press.

Smith, A. (1966) 'Speech and other functions after left (dominant) hemispherectomy,' *Journal of Neurology, Neurosurgery and Psychiatry*, 29, 467–71.

Sperry, R. W. (1962) 'Some general aspects of interhemispheric integration,' in Mountcastle, V. B. (ed.) *Interhemisheric Relations and Cerebral Dominance*, Baltimore, Md, Johns Hopkins Press, 43–9.

Sperry, R. W. (1968) 'Hemisphere deconnection and unity in conscious awareness,' *American Psychologist*, 23, 723–33.

Sperry, R. W. (1969) 'Perception in the absence of neocortical commissures,' *Research Publications of the Association of Nervous and Mental Diseases*, 48, 123–38.

Sperry, R. W. (1974) 'Lateral specialization in the surgically separated hemispheres,' in Milner, B. (ed.) *Hemispheric Specialization and Interaction*, Cambridge, Mass., MIT Press.

Stefanko, S. Z. and Schenk, V. W. D. (1979) 'Anatomical aspects of the agenesis of the corpus callosum in man,' in Russell, I. S., Van Hof, M. W. and Berlucchi, G. (eds) *Structure and Function of the Cerebral Commissures*, New York, Macmillan, 479–83.

Stein, J. (1986) 'Motor asymmetries of the cerebral hemispheres', in Rose, C. (ed) *Aphasia*, London, Churchill Livingstone (in press).

Sugishita, M., Iwata, M., Toyokura, Y., Yoshioka, M. and Yamada, R. (1978) 'Reading of ideograms and phograms in Japanese patients after partial commissurotomy,' *Neuropsychologia*, 16, 417–26.

Swanson, L. W. (1983) 'The hippocampus and the concept of the limbic system,' in Seifert, W. (ed.) *Neurobiology of the Hippocampus*, New York, Academic Press, 3–19.

Szentagothai, J. (1978a) 'The neuron network of the cerebral cortex: a functional interpretation', *Proceedings of the Royal Society of London*, B201, 219–48.

Szentagothai, J. (1978b) 'Specificity versus (quasi-)randomness in cortical connectivity,' in Brazier, M. A. B. and Petsche, H. (eds) *Architectonics of the Cerebral Cortex*, New York, Raven Press, 77–97.

Tomasch, J. (1954) 'Size, distribution and number of fibers in the human corpus callosum,' *Anatomical Record*, 119, 119–35.

Towe, A. C. (1975) 'Notes on the hypothesis of columnar organization in somatosensory cerebral cortex,' *Brain, Behavior and Evolution*, 11, 16–47.

Toyama, K., Tokashiki, S. and Matsunami, K. (1969) 'Synaptic action of commissural impulses upon association efferent cells in cat visual cortex,' *Brain Research*, 14, 518–20.

Tsao, Y., Wu, M. and Feustel, T. (1981) 'Stroop interference: hemisphere differences in Chinese speakers,' *Brain and Language*, 13, 372–8.

Tucker, D. M. (1981) 'Lateral brain function, conceptualization and emotion,' *Psychological Bulletin*, 89, 19–46.

Uttal, W. R. (1978) *The Psychobiology of Mind*, Hillsdale, NJ, Erlbaum.

von Economo, C. (1929) *The Cytoarchitectonics of the Human Cerebral Cortex*, Oxford, Oxford University Press.

Wada, J. A., Clarke, R. and Hamm, A. (1975) 'Cerebral hemispheric asymmetries in humans: cortical speech zones in 100 adult and 100 infant brains,' *Archives of Neurology*, 32, 239–46.

Waddington, C. H. (1970) 'The theory of evolution today,' in Koestler, A. and Smythies, J. R. (eds) *Beyond Reductionism*, New York, Macmillan, 357–74.

Walker, S. F. (1980) 'Lateralization of function in the vertebrate brain: a review,' *British Journal of Psychology*, 71, 329–67.

Walley, R. E. and Weiden, T. D. (1973) 'Lateral inhibition and cognitive masking: a neuropsychological theory of attention,' *Psychological Review*, 80, 284–302.

Wapner, W., Hamby, S. and Gardner, H. (1981) 'The role of the right hemisphere in the apprehension of complex linguistic materials,' *Brain and Language*, 14, 15–33.

Warren, J. M. (1977) 'Handedness and cerebral dominance in monkeys,' in Harnad, S. *et al.* (eds) *Lateralization in the Nervous System*, New York, Academic Press, 151–72.

Wasserman, G. H. (1982, 1983) 'TIMA, Parts I and II,' *Journal of Theoretical Biology*, 96, 77–86; 99, 609–28.

Webster, W. G. (1977) 'Hemispheric asymmetry in cats,' in Harnad, S. *et al.* (eds) *Lateralization in the Nervous System*, New York, Academic Press, 471–80.

Weiskrantz, L. (1979) 'On the role of cerebral commissures in animals,' in Russell, I. S. *et al.* (eds) *Structure and Function of the Cerebral Commissures*, New York, Macmillan, 475–8.

Weiskrantz, L. (1980) 'The problem of hemispheric specialization in animals,' *Pontificiae Academiae Scientiarum Scripta Varia*, 45, 573–92.

Wexler, B. E. and Henninger, G. R. (1979) 'Alterations in cerebral laterality in acute psychotic illness,' *Archives of General Psychiatry*, 36, 278–84.

Whitaker, H. A. and Ojemann, G. A. (1977) 'Lateralization of higher cortical functions: a critique,' *Annals of the New York Academy of Sciences*, 299, 459–76.

White, L. E. (1965) 'A morphologic concept of the limbic lobe,' *International Review of Neurobiology*, 8, 1–34.

Wiesel, T. N. and Hubel, D. H. (1966) 'Spatial and chromatic interactions in the lateral geniculate body of the rhesus monkey,' *Journal of Neurophysiology*, 29, 1115–56.

Winner, E. and Gardner, H. (1977) 'Comprehension of metaphor in brain-damaged patients,' *Brain*, 100, 719–27.

Wolff, J. R. and Zaborsky, L. (1979) 'On the normal arrangement of fibers and terminals and limits of plasticity in the callosal system of the rat,' in Russell, I. S. *et al.* (eds) *Structure and Function of Cerebral Commissures*, New York, Macmillan, 147–54.

Yakovlev, P. I. and Rakic, P. (1966) 'Patterns of decussation of bulbar pyramids and distribution of pyramidal tracts in two sides of the spinal cord,' *Transactions of the American Neurological Association*, 91, 366–7.

Zaidel, E. (1976) 'Auditory vocabulary of the right hemisphere following brain bisection and hemidecortication,' *Cortex*, 12, 191–211.

Zaidel, E. (1978) 'Auditory language comprehension in the right hemisphere following cerebral commissurotomy and hemispherectomy: a comparison with child language and aphasia,' in Caramazza, A. and Zurif, E. B. (eds) *Language Acquisition and Language Breakdown: Parallels and Divergences*, Baltimore, Md, Johns Hopkins Press, 229–75.

Zaidel, E. (1979) 'Performance on the TTPA following cerebral commissurotomy and hemispherectomy,' *Neuropsychologia*, 17, 259–80.

Zaidel, E. (1983) 'Advances and retreats in laterality research,' *Behavioral and Brain Sciences*, 3, 523–8.

Zaidel, E. and Sperry, R. W. (1974) 'Memory impairment after commissurotomy in man,' *Brain*, 97, 263–72.

Zimmerman, G. W. and Knott, J. R. (1974) 'Slow potentials of the brain related to speech processing in normal speakers and stutterers,' *Electroencephalography and Clinical Neurophysiology*, 37, 599–607.

Zurif, E., Caramazza, A., Myerson, R. and Galvin, J. (1974) 'Semantic feature representation for normal and aphasic language,' *Brain and Language*, 1, 167–87.

Glossary

agenesis [*a*, not + *genesis*, formation] Failure of an organ or tissue to develop during normal growth (*see* callosal agenesis).

anterior commissure [*see* commissure] The second largest forebrain commissure (one-fiftieth the size of the corpus callosum) which connects the anterior temporal lobes.

aphasia [*a*, without + *phasis*, speech] A loss of the faculty to transmit ideas using language (reading, writing, speaking and understanding speech).

axon [*axon*, axis] The essential conducting portion of a nerve fiber continuous with the cytoplasm of the nerve cell; the main output channels for neurons (*see* dendrite).

bilateral (*bi*, two + *latus*, side] Having two sides, or related to both sides (*compare* unilateral, contralateral, ipsilateral).

brain code The fundamental rules by which psychologically meaningful information is transmitted within the brain (*see* neuron code).

brainstem All parts of the brain below the cerebral hemispheres and above the spinal cord; usually divided into the upper brainstem (the thalamus and hypothalamus) and lower brainstem (midbrain, pons, cerebellum and medulla oblongata).

callosal agenesis A neurological condition in which the corpus callosum has failed to develop during fetal life.

callosumotomy [*callosum*, see corpus callosum + *-otomy*, incision] Surgical severence of the corpus callosum. The split-brain surgery.

commissure [*commissura*, bringing together or seam] A bundle of nerve fibers passing from one side to the other in the brain or spinal cord (*see* corpus callosum).

connectionism A theory of cortical function which assumes a general homogeneity of cortical structure with functional differences being primarily due to the nature of the corticocortical and cortico-brainstem connections (*compare* reductionism).

contralateral [*contra*, opposite + *latus*, side] On the opposite side (*compare* ipsilateral).

corpus callosum [*corpus*, body or mass + *callosus*, hard] The largest commissure between the cerebral hemispheres (*see* commissure).

cortical column A functional and/or structural unit of the cortex, containing 100–10,000 nerve cells – most of which show similar response characteristics.

dendrite [*dendrites*, relating to a tree] One of numerous branching cytoplasmic processes of the nerve cell; the input channels to nerve cells (*see* axon).

dichotic listening [*dicha*, in two] One of the two major means for comparing hemisphere function in normal subjects, in which different sounds are sent to the ears.

disambiguation [*dis*, separation + *ambiguus*, doubtful] The process of choosing between possible meanings of an ambiguous phrase.

dominance Usually used to mean the specialization of one hemisphere for a kind of task which presumably either hemisphere could perform, but one hemisphere is empirically found to be particularly good at. Perception of the contralateral visual field or control over the contralateral hand, etc., is not considered to be a manifestation of 'dominance,' since both hemispheres are 'dominant' for the contralateral field. Dominance effects are found, however, for speech, musical-chord recognition, etc.

dyslexia [*dys*, bad, difficult + *lexis*, word] Inability to read more than a few lines with understanding.

engram [*en*, in + *gramma*, mark] The physiological memory trace recorded in the brain. Its location and properties are unknown.

forebrain The most recently evolved part of the nervous system; subdivided into the cerebral hemispheres and the thalamus.

hemifield [*hemi*, half + field] The left or right half of the sensory field; the half of the sensory field which is recorded most strongly in the contralateral cerebral hemisphere.

hemispherectomy [*hemi*, half + *sphaira*, sphere + -*ectomy*, removal] Surgical removal of a cerebral hemisphere.

heterotopic fibers [*heteros*, other + *topos*, place] Nerve fibers which terminate at contralateral sites which are not mirror-images of their origin (*compare* homotopic fibers, symmetrical heterotopic fibers).

homotopic fibers [*homos*, same + *topos*, place] Nerve fibers which terminate at contralateral sites which are mirror-images of their origin (*compare* heterotopic fibers, symmetrical heterotopic fibers).

interhemispheric [*inter*, between + *hemi*, half + *sphaira*, sphere] Between the cerebral hemispheres.

intrahemispheric [*intra*, within + *hemi*, half + *sphaira*, sphere] Within a single cerebral hemisphere.

ipsilateral [*ipse*, self + *latus*, side] On the same side (*compare* contralateral, unilateral, bilateral).

laterality [*latus*, side] Usually used to mean lateral specialization of the cerebral hemispheres; loosely used to mean an asymmetry of specialization.

limbic lobe [*limbus*, edge, border or fringe] The phylogenetically older external rim of the cortex, generally the same as paleocortex, involved in autonomic and emotional processes and having many connections with the hypothalamus and lower brainstem.

mirror-image negative The double reversal of a two-dimensional pattern of cortical activity – a mirror-image inversion and the photographic reversal of excited and inhibited regions.

neocortex [*neo*, new + *cortex*, bark] The younger part of the outer surface of the cerebral hemispheres, thought to be involved in the highest cognitive functions (*compare* paleocortex).

neuron code The fundamental rules concerning individual neurons communicate with each other (*see* brain code).

optic chiasma [*optic*, eye + *chiasma*, crossing] The portion where the optic nerves cross over the midline. Cutting the chiasma along the midline results in all stimuli in the left visual field going to the right eye, and vice versa.

paleocortex [*palaios*, ancient + *cortex*, bark] The older portion of the cerebral cortex, generally limbic cortex (*compare* neocortex).

paralexia [*para*, near + *lexis*, speech] Misreading or the substitution of one word for another during reading.

polymodal [*poly*, many + *modus*, mode] Involving more than one sense modality (touch, vision, etc.) (*see* supramodal).

reductionism A theory of causality which, when applied to cortical functions, maintains that anatomical (usually cellular) differences between cortical areas play the predominant role in determining differences in their functional properties (*compare* connectionism).

reticular activating system A network of nerve fibers and nuclei within the brainstem whose function is to activate portions of cortex.

retinotopy [*retina*, retina + *topos*, place] The topographical representation of the pattern of retinal stimulation at various sites in the nervous system (*see also* somatotopy, tonotopy).

semantics [*semantikos* significant] The branch of linguistics concerned with meaning.

somatotopy [*soma*, body + *topos*, place] The topographical representation of body sensation found at various sites in the nervous system (*see also* retinotopy, tonotopy).

somesthetic [*soma*, body + *aisthesis*, sensation] Somatosensory; referring to bodily sensation or the sense of touch.

stereopsis [*stereos*, solid + *opsis*, vision] The ability to see the three-dimensionality of solid objects, due to the combining of slightly different viewpoints from the eyes.

supramodal [*supra*, above + *modus*, mode] Abstract information processing which is not directly related to any of the sense modalities (*see* polymodal).

symmetrical heterotopic fibers Fibers which terminate at sites which are not mirror-images of their origin, but which have mirror-image fibers in the contralateral hemisphere.

tachistoscope [*tachistos*, most rapid + *skopeo*, to examine] Instrument used for rapid presentation of visual stimuli usually to the left or right half of the retina to compare the recognition thresholds of the cerebral hemispheres (etc.).

thalamus [*thalamos*, bed or bedroom] A major relay station for all sensory stimuli except olfaction; contains both specific (relay) nuclei and nonspecific nuclei involved in associational and attentional processes.

tonotopy [*tonos*, pitch + *topos*, place] The topographical representation of sound frequencies at various sites in the nervous system (*see also* retinotopy, somatotopy).

topographical [*topos*, place + *graphe*, description] Of or relating to the two-dimensional patterning of cortical activity.

unilateral [*uni*, one + *latus*, side] Having or pertaining to one side only (*compare* bilateral, contralateral, ipsilateral).

Index